Crooked Angels

Carol Lee is an author, journalist and Alexander Technique teacher. She is a visiting lecturer in journalism at the Department of Postgraduate Studies, City University, London and has written for the *Observer, Independent, Guardian, Sunday Times,* and many national magazines.

Her play, *Feet First,* was staged at the King's Head, Islington, London

Crooked Angels is her sixth book.

ALSO BY CAROL LEE

The Ostrich Position
Friday's Child
The Blind Side of Eden
Talking Tough
Good Grief

Crooked Angels

Carol Lee

ARROW

Published by Arrow Books in 2002

3 5 7 9 10 8 6 4 2

Copyright © Carol Lee 2001

Carol Lee has asserted her right under the Copyright, Designs and
Patents Act, 1988 to be identified as the author of this work

First published in the United Kingdom in 2001 by Century
Arrow Books Limited
The Random House Group Limited
20 Vauxhall Bridge Road, London SW1V 2SA

Random House Australia (Pty) Limited
20 Alfred Street, Milsons Point, Sydney,
New South Wales 2061, Australia

Random House New Zealand Limited
18 Poland Road, Glenfield,
Auckland 10, New Zealand

Random House South Africa (Pty) Ltd
Endulini, 5a Jubilee Road, Parktown 2193, South Africa

Random House UK Limited Reg. No. 954009

www.randomhouse.co.uk

A CIP record for this book is available
from the British Library

Papers used by Random House UK Limited are natural,
recyclable products made from wood grown in sustainable
forests. The manufacturing processes conform to the
environmental regulations of the country of origin.

ISBN 0 09 941612 3

Typeset in Fairfield by
MATS, Southend-on-Sea, Essex

Printed and bound in Great Britain by
Bookmarque Ltd, Croydon, Surrey

To the grandparents:

Harry and Bessie (née Theodocia);
Nellie and Owen

Contents

Acknowledgements

I would like to thank:

Sandy and Peter, who were steadfast and refused to be frightened; my brother, Chris, for his encouragement and support; Laura Longrigg at MBA for being a marvellous agent; Sue for housing me; Renzo Molinari for his skill and intuition; Gillian McCredie, who read the drafts of this; Dr J W Scadding, Consultant Neurologist, Whittington Hospital, London; Hannah Black at Century; Martin Western for trips to the seaside, a return to Kenya, and African pictures.

I would also like to thank Ivy Scott for family stories; her late husband, Alf, who made log fires on winter's nights; the Society of Authors' Francis Head Awards and the Royal Literary Fund for generous assistance at the time of writing.

Chapter One

~§

PIECES OF A PERSON

The deep part of my story, the spine of it, goes back more than a century to the mid-1890s, to an eight-year-old girl sitting on a suburban train, clutching a rough bundle in her arms.

The bundle is heavy. It contains folded mailbags and factory sewing, the coarse material and weight of which have bled her mother's fingers – and will do worse to her.

Sitting still on the train, she doesn't want anyone to know about the coins in the cloth pouch under her skirt, money for her mother.

But I shall begin a hundred years or more after these journeys. Here, in a different part of London, a woman is about to wake up.

It's 6.30 and bright, the beginning of a high summer's day. Moving to get up, I reach towards the nearby window to open the curtains and, as my feet touch the ground, it happens. There's something badly wrong with my head. Heavy as a waterlogged football, it will pull me face down to the floor if I let it. And what's happened to my neck? Why can't it hold my head? For a moment I daren't move. Then, in slow motion, bring down my arm from where it was reaching to let in the light.

None of the neighbourhood sounds have started up yet: loud music from the house next door; barking dog in the garden next to that. But my mind is busy. I'm scanning my body: counting; adding up symptoms; recording; as if facts would make me safe.

Pins and needles. Ah, but only in my left hand and only in three fingers. Did I wake up like that? Yes. Can I wiggle them? Yes, but slowly. They don't feel personal: they're like things attached to me. Why's that? Shall I get a pin? No, it might be dangerous, the way I'm trembling.

Walking towards the bathroom, my arms, legs, head, spine are separate, no communication between parts. The thread or piece of elastic which keeps a body joined up has gone. Something is missing from my spine.

In the bathroom mirror, I look the same. No swollen-headedness, no abnormality on the surface, but pieces of me are strangers to each other: hands, feet, arms, legs.

My neck kept still and my head upright for fear I'll lose it, I get dressed, go to the study and sit down at the keyboard. Switching on the computer, part of me is terrified and another part calm. The calm part won't accept I can't work. It's what I do, get up in the morning and write. It's what I've done for years and am doing now to defend myself against the nightmare.

For a few minutes I tap in words and pretend this is a normal morning. Then the pain begins. It starts in my forearms, like a heavy ache, and, within minutes, my arms are trapped, gripped in what feels like a pair of steel vices. They squeeze deeper until there's no life left in me from my elbows to the tips of my fingers. The 'breath' has been squeezed from my arms.

But I still won't accept what is happening. It's what you read about in books or newspapers. It happens out there, to other people, and it can't be here. It mustn't be. I can't let it. I move to lift an arm in protest, to dismiss what is happening to me and brush it away, but I'm met with a locked shoulder joint. My arm won't move. It can't be shifted. It's heavy and lifeless like a dead object in my lap.

Panic. I have never been disabled. I have walked, run, danced, played tennis, moved freely and now I'm shut in, my body betraying me. Swift on panic, retreat begins, an attempt to escape. Looking up, seconds later, I've moved light years away from the world outside. I can see and hear it from my seat at the desk, but I can't feel it. Invisible glass panels have slid silently shut around me. Sealed off in a dome-like bubble, sounds from the street are far away. Doors shutting, cars moving, children calling are all there, but where am I?

Cut off from the outside world, I'm remote, too, from my body, made up of pieces now, bits of a person. On top of my body there's this waterlogged skull which is not my normal head. Useless arms hang from my side and I can't trust my spine. Though still in the same skin, I'm no longer at home. Something in the middle of me, whatever links bodies and keeps them acting as a whole, has been stolen in the night.

These are the physical symptoms, or, the start of them. They get worse and more varied and one of them, the electric shock, will bring me to my knees. But this particular pain hasn't happened yet. There are still a number of hours to go.

There's a swivel chair in the bay window and maybe I'll be safe if I can get to it. Once there, I fall into a long, strange sleep.

Waking two or three hours later, I seem drugged. Anchored to the back of my seat, I can't find the power or will to lift myself. So I don't and most of the day takes place without me. From late morning to afternoon to early evening I sit looking out of the window, only my eyelids moving every now and then with a slow blink. I'm unconcerned about anything at all. Wherever the strange sleep took me, it changed something and I think I will probably find no reason to move again. I shall stay in the chair for ever.

Finding the strength at last I move, as in a trance, downstairs to the kitchen. Reaching slowly to open a cupboard door, what feels like a high-voltage electric charge flashes – or judders – through the length of my arm. This is it. The electric shock has arrived and the pain is unbearable. It's gone within seconds, but the shadow of it remains like a deep bruise under my skin. My arm feels beaten, done for, and I don't want the shock to come back. The pain would drive me mad.

So this is the beginning of the story told in my body. I go to bed as the woman I am: an author, playwright, journalist, lecturer. I have friends, a house, health. I play the piano, play tennis, swim, dance, hold parties. By the time I wake up in the morning, this description of my life isn't true any more.

Chapter Two

৽

THE BIG GUNS

Walking to the surgery the next day, I could be drunk. My sleep the previous night had seemed drugged again and I stay close to walls, brushing along hedges and fences, lightly touching gates. I believe I sway and tilt and am afraid of falling over. Yet I am walking straight. The lurching is inside where a fault line has opened up, a crack in the ground. The feeling from the previous morning, that parts of me don't belong to each other, is now real. They don't.

My GP away, I see someone else. A 'trapped nerve' is what it sounds like to her and a neck X-ray arranged for the following day. She explains what she thinks is wrong, says that nerves fan out into the body from the spinal cord. The ones which run through arms come from the top of the spine – the neck. Maybe there's a problem, here, with a disc and it's trapping a nerve, causing pain and the rest of the havoc that's going on.

The X-ray result brings relief, first of all, when it's clear, but not for long. If it isn't a trapped nerve, then what is it? Whatever's wrong has to be sorted out quickly, for I'm quietly desperate. I am not myself. The problem is urgent.

And it stays that way.

It's summer. Different doctors coming and going off on holiday offer advice, none of it the same. One recommends osteopathy. Another is against it. One tells me to rest, another to keep moving as much as I can. Yet another says the problem is probably muscular and may take a long time to sort itself out.

No one knows what's wrong with me.

Over the next few months, five different GPs, three osteopaths, three physiotherapists and an acupuncturist all have ideas about what's happening inside my body. All are different. A trapped nerve, too much tennis, inflammation in the brachial plexus, tendonitis, a frozen shoulder muscle, a mystery disease. Some say the problem is in the arms; others that it's in the neck.

Tested for relevant possibilities, from carpel tunnel syndrome to rheumatoid arthritis to MS, there are still no answers, only baffling offers of different cures. I need a cortisone injection, a series of arm-manipulations, bed rest, an adjustment to my spine, or a collar to be worn at all times, even at night. The hospital doctor suggesting this says it will prevent wear and tear on my neck. Someone else says it will wither the muscles. It's up to me what I do – but what if I make the wrong choice?

Attending a hospital physiotherapy department for the first time, a woman there is sympathetic to my bewilderment at being healthy one minute and stricken the next and I believe she will make me better. Young and competent-looking, with short fair hair and a still, serious manner, her calmness reassures me. She asks detailed questions and says she will work to relieve tightness in nerve channels when we next meet. This will stop the pain.

Preparing for the next session, showering and dressing slowly, as I must, I can barely contain my excitement. Someone knows what's wrong at last. This treatment will work and the nightmare will soon be over. I'll be well within weeks, enter the tennis tournament, ring my doubles partner, say I'm ready to defend the title we won last year.

Lying me on my back, the physiotherapist moves my spine and legs in different positions and tests my arms as she does so, turning them gently at first, and then pulling them slowly to see when they hurt. They're numb in some positions, painful in others. I don't mind this if the treatment will cure me. But that night, my arms are alive, searing with relentless pain. There's nowhere I can be, on my back, front, side, without them throbbing, burning, aching.

Sunrise finds me in the swivel chair in the study,

arms resting in pillows on my lap. They look peaceful now, palms open, fingers lightly curled. But at some godforsaken hour of the night I'd wanted them chopped off. I'd have given away my arms to a passing axe man, anything to be rid of the pain. I can't stand another night like this. I'll have to remain untreated, at least for a while.

Going it alone for the next few weeks, the pain seems to be triggered by movement in the upper half of my body: reaching for a towel, bending forwards, turning round. Like a detective shadowing a suspect, I try to second-guess the pain. Watching out for it, moving slowly, being still and alert at the same time, I see if I can catch it before it catches me, find where it comes from – and why.

When I arrive for hospital tests some of the people who examine me are flummoxed by how healthy I look. Tennis, walking, swimming have made me fit. But close questioning reveals an intermittent pain behind the top of my right shoulder. I'd put it down to my tennis serve – heavy and flat. Doctors go 'Ah-ha' in a slow way when I tell them about it, but they're still no nearer sorting out what's wrong. The tests reveal normal reflexes, good muscle tone, an athlete's pulse, steady heartbeat, good eyesight, enviable blood pressure. Nothing else.

Stalled in this way, in a kind of limbo of half-grief, I mourn what I can't do and am grateful for what I can.

But how long can I go on avoiding people? Friends, neighbours, family are used to my busyness, to my being away at times, travelling for work, or hiding at home, planning a new book. They are also used to me coming back – and I've been 'gone' for weeks now.

As the summer goes on, I push way under, out of sight and mind, the fact that I can't work and am self-employed with a mortgage to pay.

The list of what I *can* do, I build on. So long as I move slowly and carefully I can bathe, dress, use a knife and fork, nudge open doors, turn a key in a lock and walk short distances. So long as I stay close to walls, hedges, trees and gateposts, I can go out. But opening things is laborious: a purse; handbag; envelope; milk carton; bottle; desk drawer; lid of a jar.

On good days, I know how daft it is to fear my head will roll off the top of my body if I don't hang on to it. On bad days, I'm nearly defeated by the amount of self-conscious effort it takes to go for a short walk. Exhausted from the struggle of holding myself together on the one hand and fending off pain with the other, the swivel chair in the study is my main daytime retreat. I lie back, head resting, arms cradled; still, except for my eyes watching the street.

Sensing, by this time, whatever is wrong won't kill me, I wonder, though, if I will recover from it and what kind of life there will be if I don't. Small things bother me – like making a cup of coffee. Watching every movement of lifting an arm, turning on a tap, filling a kettle, picking up a jar, unscrewing the lid, opening a drawer, fetching a spoon, it takes so long, so much attention to detail. Then, when the coffee is ready, I can't lift the mug to my lips. The first stab of the electric shock warns me my arm-use is up for now. I must rest — for ten minutes, half an hour or the whole day, whatever it takes.

I learn a trick. By putting the mug on a high enough surface, I can drink without bending my body forwards too much. It means standing up, but it's better than nothing. Sometimes there's triumph in this. I *will* have my coffee. There's humour even. It takes two or three different surface heights to drink most of it without clasping the mug in my hands, or bending too much, so I get a tour of the house: I start at the mantelpiece, go on to a bookshelf and end up on the piano.

Leaning towards the piano lid drinking coffee one day, the warmth of the summer reveals other un-welcome guests — intruders in the basement of my house. I spot their tendrils on the skirting board which crumbles away like powder in my hand. The floorboards are up within days. Living room turned into a hole in the ground, the builders call me to see what they've found at the bottom.

They're big as dinner plates and lifelike as octopuses. Giant mushrooms. Rot growing. I'm almost sick at the sight of their huge, bloated bodies. They've flourished because there's rubble where there should have been space under the house for air to pass through.

Gathering damp over the years, this old pile of earth and stones has been food for the triffids.

Arms cradled against the pain, all I can do is look – but how far have their tentacles reached? Is the whole lower part of the house affected? Has the rot – dry and wet are both flourishing – crept up the stairs? Is my house, like my body, on the verge of collapse?

I'm told the bill to fix it will be big. I resist my first impulse: to have everything put back together again and pretend there's nothing wrong. Even with chemical spraying under the floorboards, will I be able to trust the house now, I wonder? Will a rogue tentacle, like a cancer cell, be missed in the dark and left to multiply?

I have fears about hidden tentacles in my body too, about the stringy network of nerves which brings pain to my arms, head, neck.

By the time two men arrive to knock down the rest of what was once my living room, the decision has taken place. I'll move. With money running out, I won't be able to meet the bills much longer. I'll sell this three-storey Victorian terraced home, put the piano in storage, pay off the mortgage, buy a smaller place – and time to recover.

Sitting in a chair on the top floor, pains strafing and shooting through my arms, I fall into another of my heavy daytime sleeps. To the sound of sledgehammers pounding in the rooms below, I dream of battlefields, wounded bodies and trying to escape from the war, but

I can't get away from gunshots and the searing flashes in my arms.

Hours later, waking from this, I give the pains in my arms a name, the Big Guns. I see them as a pair of steel-eyed cannons. Swivelling round together, they search for their target, and I'm helpless in between.

I must get out of this. I must do something.

Chapter Three

HANNAH

Arriving at Hannah's consulting rooms on a crisp, fine autumn morning, it's six weeks since the mushrooms have been shovelled off the bare earth underneath my basement floorboards and four months since the Big Guns took me hostage. For many hours a day I sit cradling my arms to fend them off. Resting back against the study chair, I think they can't spot me when I'm still. It's when I move I'm a target. Non-resting times are spent trying to sell the house, keeping hospital and doctors' appointments and reassuring friends I'm managing.
I'm not.

Fear of the pain – and doing anything that will make it flare – has stilled me down, almost to nothing. I've taken myself away, retreated a long way back from where the surface of my skin meets the air outside me. Tucked down like this, snail-sized, where the Guns can't find me, I wait.

—

Hannah is a physiotherapist who specialises in sports injuries. She was found through a phone call to a friend, a man who woke one morning to find he could barely move a muscle. Within weeks, she caused him to pick up his bed and walk, and he's been fit ever since. He's full of praise for her:

'I'll give her a gold-plated reference,' he says, giving me her number.

She is one of the people who believes the cause of the problem lies in the neck. Her way of dealing with this is through mechanical traction: sessions which involve stretching my neck and spine on a contraption which looks like an instrument of torture.

During treatments I lie on my back, chin cupped in a cloth pouch attached by straps to a pulley-type mechanism standing behind my head. When the machine starts up, weights at the top of it drop down, tautening the straps, pulling my neck and stretching my spine. The pull on my body then releases as the weights go up and begins again as they descend. The treatment goes on for four or five minutes.

I later learn how this kind of traction is commonly used in hospitals and private consulting rooms. Two crucial factors are: the angle of the neck in relation to the machine (they must be in a straight line); the amount of weight in the pulley. Conventional wisdom says a neck, the most delicate part of the spine, shouldn't be 'pulled' with more than 10 per cent of the patient's bodyweight.

I don't know this at the time. Nor do I know that like many other treatments, surgery for example, mechanical traction is high risk if not expertly used.

But it isn't Hannah's expertise I'm concerned about to begin with. It's her strange behaviour, the way she keeps on looking at herself in a floor-length mirror in her consulting room, even talking to me through her reflection in the glass. If I'm standing up with my back to it, she finds herself in the mirror over my shoulder.

Gold-plated reference aside, what am I doing trusting my neck to her? The reason is clear. After three or four sessions, there's improvement: I can turn my neck, and this feels like a small miracle to a woman who's been sitting in an armchair for the last four months. If Hannah can get me well again, I'll have to take her as she is.

Then, one afternoon, after about eight sessions, Hannah's impatience gets the better of her. Or something does. As she chats away and peruses herself in the looking glass on the wall, she decides to speed things up a bit. She puts 7 kilos of weights on the traction machine instead of the 3 kilos she usually uses.

I am 57 kilos. Not that she's asked. I realise later Hannah hasn't asked my weight, age, address or taken more than a few sketchy details about me. There's no medical history written down. Maybe it wouldn't have made any difference. But the traction does. It would take a bulldozer to shift some people's necks. Seven kilos does for mine.

Getting up off the couch, I'm okay, but by later in the day there's a persistent – and peculiar – headache. It spreads upwards like a thick column of steel-plated ants marching from the back of my neck, through my scalp and up over the top of my head. The headache doesn't go when I sleep that night, nor all the following day. It's accompanied by something else – difficulty in swallowing.

On the phone, Hannah tells me to come back to see her.

'Ah,' she says when we're face to face. 'Traction sometimes gives you a small headache. Come here and I will take it away for you.

'Don't concern yourself,' she says as the pulley goes up and down. 'The problem with swallowing will disappear in a few days.'

It doesn't. Instead, I begin to choke on food, and there's a flickering in the corners of my eyes, like a TV on the blink. I phone the optician.

'Your eyes are okay,' he reassures me. 'But have you got a bad headache?'

I tell him about the traction.

'Don't have any more,' he says firmly, 'and go and see your GP.'

At the surgery, painkillers are all that's on offer and I daren't take them for fear of being addicted to anything that will shift the ant army off my skull.

In the weeks which follow, hindsight torments me: Why? Why did I let her do it? Why didn't I follow my instincts all along? Why was I so stupid? Why oh why did I let her give me traction again? Why didn't I sit down *then* and protest?

I've been suffering what is known in the medical profession as a traction headache for ten days when I confront Hannah. The meeting is terse. Some of the previous week has been spent in the library and I've made phone calls, the most disturbing to a man at the tennis club. He's been seeing a physio for a back problem. Has he had traction himself I ask.

'No way,' he says. 'My best friend's wife was practically crippled by it. She went in with a small pain in her neck, and came out in a hell of a state. That was a year ago, and she's never been right since. She's in permanent pain and no one can help her. I wouldn't touch traction with a barge pole. Don't do it.'

'Why did you do it?' I ask Hannah, a few days later.

She's done it to try and speed things up she says. She knew I needed to work. She knew I'd been 'sick' a long time. She was doing it for me.

I'm having none of it.

Then she admits: 'I should not have done it the second time, after you said you had the headache. It was the second treatment that was the problem.' But realising what she's just owned up to, she then goes back on herself:

'It should not last this long, you know, this headache. If it stays, the problem is in the neck, not in the treatment.'

So there. It's the neck's fault, not hers. And a neck

can only prove its innocence – or otherwise – if you cut it open.

Walking away from Hannah's consulting rooms where I had gone with such hope, trust is fast receding and me with it. The world outside is a long way off from where I'm stranded deep inside myself. It's a beautiful, crisp late autumn day; sights and sounds are sharp, traffic and the world roaring by, none of it reaching me.

My reflection in windows doesn't say who I am any more. At home, my face in the mirror doesn't describe me. I'm like a frozen black and white snapshot of who I once was. I try and imagine a time when I might return to life and not be a stranger; when I might step back into the outside world, competent, animated and unresentful. The trees are still there, and the buildings, and perhaps they'll wait and perhaps one day I won't have a headache.

In the weeks after confronting Hannah, cracks in my perception open up. My sense of perspective is out of true; my mind and body are giving me two different versions of reality. To my mind, a walk round the park is a good idea; to my body it's an assault course, with bumps and dips like potholes. Thinking I've lurched into a crater, I turn to look and there's nothing there but a slight unevenness in the path. Yet I used to run round this park, local schoolboys joshing me for the uncool way I raced flat out. Other times, I think I'm falling over while I'm standing up. But is this a figment of my body's imagination, or my mind's?

There are further problems with my daily comings and goings outside the house. I look physically normal, but I'm not, and people don't understand.

Waiting at a bus stop, arms in their usual cradling place, my hands folded loosely on top of them, a teenage girl next to me lifts her baby out of his pushchair from where he's been smiling at us both. With the bus approaching, she wants to fold up the buggy, and passes me the baby.

'I can't,' I say as he dangles, legs kicking, between us. 'My arms don't work.' But they do up to a point, and I look so reliable.

There's a woman in her seventies who lives in the area. Going blind, she gets by through asking for people's arms to lean on from time to time. It's only arms she wants: for crossing roads; getting on buses; negotiating rough ground, and she's leant on mine before. Recognising my voice, she wants an arm and wonders why I won't let her have it.

On days when I feel daring, or just plain bloody-minded, I still go out, but it gets more difficult. A bad shot of pain would change me in an instant from a woman holding on to herself into one who is not.

Time and again I come back to the missing thread in my spine, the stolen piece of elastic in my backbone, like a screw missing in a mind. It haunts me. How long can a sane woman shelter inside a mad, un-remembering body?

Chapter Four

ॐई

A MINIATURE WOMAN

Winter approaching, the chasm between where I am on the inside and who I am to the outside world widens. I'm running two versions of a life, the one on the surface where I appear almost normal and the interior one where I'm marooned in my body like a small island in a vast sea. To keep going, I have to manage the gap between the two. So as not to get caught out, I trim down activities. Work is jettisoned. So is cleaning the house, playing the piano, attending meetings, entertaining friends, swimming, cleaning shoes, sewing on buttons, carrying shopping bags, drinking coffee, holding babies and catching buses.

I eke out my daily quota of arm-use before the Big Guns discover I'm out and about and come to get me. Behaving like Scrooge, I become mean with what little movement I have left in the upper part of my body. It's a small life I'm leading.

So much of me gone, it's awkward with people now. I don't wash up when friends cook for me. I don't do anything for anybody any more, and more and more I keep myself away and withdraw because the difference in me – past and present – is too big to get over. I can't bear seeing it in friends' eyes. Why won't I be better? is the unspoken question between us.

Why won't I be who – and how – I was before? Why won't I be funny again, arrange things for people, organise days out, laugh the way I used to, or answer the phone? Where have I gone? And – it's been months now – will I come back?

They can't believe what's happening to me and they won't accept there isn't an answer: 'Have you tried so and so?' they ask, rifling through address books. 'He worked wonders for a woman in my office when she could barely move with pain.'

'Why don't you try another doctor? Look, this friend of mine saw this man in Harley Street and she only went to him twice and . . .'

'Let me find out the name of the physio who cured the man upstairs . . .'

Then there are entreaties. Have I tried different kinds of treatments? What about a chiropractor? Have I thought of shiatsu, massage, reflexology? I don't tell them the story of why I won't try anyone else. I hardly credit it myself: that a string of people in white coats haven't helped; that for months I've joined hospital queues, had tests, visited all kinds of practitioners and failed to be better.

I long for someone with a magic wand, a cross between the best doctor in the world and a fairy godmother, but that's how I found Hannah. I'm still trying to recover from her treatment. I choke on food, have difficulty swallowing and the upper part of my body is in a self-imposed straitjacket. She was the seventh or eighth practitioner I'd seen, and I'd got her from a friend. The hospital physiotherapist I saw before her made me worse too, and other people have added small pains: stinging nettle sensations, tennis elbow twinges, aching neck muscles, the feeling of flames fanning along my arms.

The man at the tennis club rings to say his friend's wife, the woman who had traction the previous year, has committed suicide. He's phoning, he says, just to add to his advice to me not to do it. Too late, for me as well as her. I don't want to think about what drove her to kill herself and how trapped she might have felt.

But if I refuse treatment, go it alone again, I won't know how to check things. What, who will be my pain-ometer? There are so many small pains by now, I can't work out from one hour, or week, to the next whether an arm, a hand, a shoulder is better or worse. Where will my sense of direction lie — in my mind or my body? Who will keep me safe?

Around this time, November, a woman called Sue — tall, fair, early forties — decides, on the spot, to buy my house:

'I'll have it,' she says, within minutes of crossing my doorstep. 'It's just what I want.'

Sue has three jobs, three cats – or is it four? – and there's a catch to the purchase. She wants to move in straight away. In a long chain which will collapse if she doesn't let her buyer in, she makes me an offer. If I let her move in the day we sign the contract, I can stay on as an unofficial tenant in two rooms, my study and bedroom, till I find somewhere – and can have the run of the house when she's out. She will be out a lot, she tells me, 'So we shan't be in each other's way.'

Being a tenant in a property I once owned brings the dangerous sensation I'm losing sight of myself altogether. What's happening in the house is too close to what's happening in my body. Even my voice sounds different. Seemingly loud, and echoing in the space inside me, I don't like it. Startled by its loudness, I stop speaking, or suddenly lower it;

'What did you say?' someone asks on the end of the phone. 'Say that again. I can't hear you.'

Resting by day in my study, head back in the high swivel chair, sometimes I'm being swept away inside myself, a canoe down a river. Whether sitting or standing, the feeling of being carried off is powerful, yet I haven't moved an inch. Other times it's slightly different: my life's an ocean with the miniature version of me drifting in it, floating in the winter sea my body has become to me.

Then there are times I'm going under, sinking through layers, diving or plummeting through deep water. The torrent, the noise and clamour of my life, is all interior – and shadowy. There must be a logical reason for this, but while the head on top of my shoulders is holding fast and thinking as best it can, a current is threatening to sweep me off.

Spending hours like this in the armchair, I wonder are the Big Guns driving me mad or was I mad before I met them? I want to continue believing in myself and in my place in a world I can no longer feel, but when I close my eyes, a film sequence comes. It's something from an old black and white picture: a woman hanging from a window ledge by her fingertips; beneath her, swirling waters.

Here, indoors, there are cats for company. One of them spits and hisses at anything which moves and clouts the others round the ear when she gets the chance. She was once feral – 'What do you mean "once"?' I ask their owner.

I look forward to Sue coming home: hearing news of her day in the outside world; a glass of wine in front of the telly; a chat about the cats' misdemeanours. But I'm allergic to them, and to keep from suffering swollen eyes and stuffed-up nostrils, I close my bedroom and study doors. They object, and hold regular protest meetings outside my bedroom – usually at around 2 a.m. I wake to hear their thumps, caterwauls and scamperings up and down the stairway.

By day, I feed this tribe; take in masses of post for a famous actress for whom Sue works as one of her three jobs; let the various people who deliver post know that 'No, the famous actress doesn't live on the premises' – so autographs are not in the offing; keep the kitchen surfaces clean – I am capable of that much; and look at smaller and smaller properties. My dream home is shrinking, as I am. To get a mortgage you need to be working, and I'm five months into incapacity.

Yet I can't bear to see another physiotherapist or osteopath. I'm frightened of being touched. Just beneath the skin, the pain waits, near the surface. I freeze when a friend moves to hug me.

Sitting so many hours in the chair, past images and incidents begin to crowd in on me – especially from Africa. I recall how, as a child living in the bush, I had seen trapped animals, deer or antelope mostly. I think of the day a young impala caught itself in some loose barbed wire from our garden fence. It lay kicking and struggling, the wire biting deeper into it. Standing helplessly nearby I tried, with my child's mind, to will it into stillness.

I attempt the same for myself now, willing myself not to struggle, not to tug against the wire.

At times I want to pick up the tennis racquet and swing it hard so my hurting arms fly off my body. Then, it's switching on the computer and typing till I kill my arms that way. When this kind of 'arm murder' is on my mind, I go back to the chair, retreating from the fury, drifting under.

There's a goldfish in the study at this time. It belongs to a neighbour's five-year-old daughter who has asked me to take care of it while she goes on holiday. Before she leaves I discuss with her the tricky business of the fish's possible demise in my custody:

'What if it dies while you're away?' I ask her. 'I can feed it and keep it company for you, but I don't want you being cross with me when you get back.'

Looking at the fish, I think I too am in a bowl of sorts, and like the creature there, I could open my mouth against the glass and no sound would come out.

But something is happening in my dreams. The cats' commotions outside the bedroom can't compete with the animals in my sleep – zebra, hundreds of them. There's movement and fear. Large herds are restless and ready to run: zebra wheeling round in a tight band, treading the ground, shaking their heads, stamping their feet, about to break loose. Round and round they go, a circle of stripes. The dreams are the same, hot dusty African plains, clouds of red earth, taut striped bodies. They wheel and stay; wheel and stay.

By day, sitting half awake, half asleep, the landscape from another part of an African childhood comes back – the swimming pool in Tanzania, and my teenage love affair with diving. Dozens of times a day I would dive: a slow run along the board; an easy slip through the water; surging under the surface to the other end; a haul out and measured walk back. Then the same all over again. I was OD'ing on warm sun in a vast African sky, cool water, high plateau air, laughter, freedom, ease.

Sitting in the armchair, dizzy with dreams, I find myself replicating this dive, falling into myself without being able to stop it. Down, down I go, fingertips first, through the middle of the sea my body has become. Head forward, back straight, ankles together, it's as if the years have rolled away and let me slip through.

Now, the outside of me, where my skin meets the world, is as far away as the top of a wave is to the seabed. I've gone and arrived at the same time. I'm relieved, first of all, to be rid of the pain, and also afraid. If this is madness, will I find my way back?

But it can't be. Madness is bedlam, chaos, betrayal and this isn't. It seems I have arrived, at last, at the bottom of myself, a place so vast you would never want to be on top again. It's limitless and here, on the ocean floor, sorrow and grief have no place. Nor the woman who typed a thousand words before breakfast.

There are no more anxious dreams at night: animals swirling in the dust, poised for flight in a barred circle. There's a place, instead, of no restraint, sleep a pacific parent – and me?

Time parts, and like a fish or a sea-snake, I slip through the hours and the years.

Chapter Five

MY MOTHER'S VOICE

In the armchair, diving in the sea of my body, I return to a time when my mother, my father and myself lived in a suburban flat in Sanderstead, Surrey. It's on the ground floor of a house converted into three fair-sized apartments. The stairway connecting these separate homes is used by everyone, and I spend much of my time on it.

I'm four, a sociable child, hanging round the hallway and staircase, waiting for someone to pass by to say hello to. I am liberal with my hellos both inside and outside the house, often getting my mother into trouble on our daily walks together. Young, pretty and shy of strangers, men soon discover how to approach her.

'Would you like a piece of chocolate?' a local widower says, bending towards me.

'Ooh, yes please,' I say with a nod which sets my ringlets bouncing.

Sometimes the chocolate is at this man's house, and I tug my mother along to his door. Then I find we walk the other way to the shops, the long way round, so we don't pass his home any more.

Brought up in a small Welsh mining village where everyone knows each other, my mother finds England and speaking English difficult. Welsh is her first language. Her husband, my daddy, is often away working and she finds this difficult too. He comes back at weekends, but sometimes his work is too far away.

We are a pair of good girls, my mother and me and, as a treat, once a month we go to London, catching the bus to Croydon and then a tram to the middle of the City. There we walk, from St Paul's Cathedral to Trafalgar Square to see the pigeons, from the Houses of Parliament to Buckingham Palace to see the Queen. We have cocoa and cake in a Lyons corner house and wherever we go there are trams, cars, shops, people and things to see.

It never matters if the Queen is out, as long as my mother, the Queen I love best in the world, is holding my hand in hers. Both our backs are straight as we walk along, looking at things everywhere we go. It's a good time to be a child. Born after the war has ended, no bombs in my head, no destruction. Shops and houses are being built as London is put back together again.

When I brush my teeth before going to bed at night, I think of all the new things I've seen and the pictures they make in my mind. Sometimes I try and count how much we saw today, how many trams we went on and the people who smiled at us in shops.

The first shadow over these brimful days happens here. Although I love my daddy, I belong to my mother. I know this because of the way she smiles at me – and her voice. Her smile goes all over my body – a warm feeling – and her voice pulls me back to her from where I play, sometimes, at the bottom of the garden. It's deep, with shadows, waves and echoes in it, and we're joined, my mother and me, by its musical strings.

My mother speaks slowly in English and I listen to her carefully, as I'm told I must. I listen out too. She doesn't want to call me twice. When she speaks Welsh she talks fast, but my father and his mother, Nana Lee, don't understand Welsh, so I don't learn any in case I say it by mistake. I'm nervous of saying things by mistake and sometimes I practise on my dolls, speaking slowly like my mother:

'Now . . . you . . . sit . . . there . . .'

Then, my mother begins to lose her English words. They get too heavy for her. Shaking her head and holding her hand to her throat, she bends forward to point things out to me, but she doesn't say them any more. I begin to be lost and afraid without her words. Fetching stories from her lap, I would bring them back to a place where I could turn and shine them; add them on to how much I already knew. Now her lap is empty.

You have to be very quiet when someone is having a nervous breakdown in your house, and that's what's happening to my mother. My father away so much, the house goes cold to me, and the world at the bottom of the garden is cold too. Without the strings from my mother's voice, I'm afraid to go there to play. I think my mother will be gone when I get back.

Our walks together and going-out times stop because my mother loses all her shiny hair: alopecia. It starts coming away in lumps and soon there's none left. She sits in the chair with her head turned away from me. There's a loud silence with no sentences in it. I can't find my mother's voice, and I'm not allowed to look for it.

My mother's hair grows back when we go to live in Wales for a while, strong and shiny as it was before. But before this, on one of his visits, my father tells me my mother is poorly and I have to be quiet. I mustn't ask questions, bother her or be a nuisance. If I want her to stay with me, and not go to a hospital where I won't see her, I must be a very good girl indeed and play by myself the best I can. If I make a noise, my mother will go away, and it will be my fault. I must be careful not to do this. So I wait for her to be better again, and it's a long time.

Early in the morning, I go and play on the stairs. Without making a noise, I crawl up on my stomach to the next flat and lie trying to see through the crack under the door or curled round pretending to be a cat. Then I come down slowly with my nose first, looking over the top of the carpet to see what's there. My head feels big and empty and I want to fill it up with sounds.

I say words to myself, softly, to keep them alive.

I mustn't slide on the bannisters, but I hold them tight, and run fingers between the bars, poking my nose round, pushing and twisting arms and legs through to the other side.

My imagination is enormous. I make up animals and soldiers, people and places, and visits to toy shops. I believe if I shut my eyes tight on the stairs I will open them to find everything I have made a wish for come true: talking dolls; noisy soldiers, parties, people, circuses, sounds, Buckingham Palace and Trafalgar Square.

Sometimes relatives come to stay from Wales, and my mother is happy and talks fast again. But it's not the same as in my wishes. There are no other children in those and when the grown-ups' backs are turned a girl cousin and myself argue over a teddy bear.

'It's mine.'

'I want to play with it.'

'You can't.'

We stand, her at one end of it, me at the other, pulling.

When the visitors go away I want to know how long till the next time they come and how many days it is. My mother wraps Time up in parcels for me, like presents, and says I have to wait till I can open them. But I want things to happen now. I want to open my presents, and I push and shove hard on hours and days trying to rip them open.

Time is too long now, and I don't like it. I want it to happen faster. I go to bed at six o'clock, and it's eight or nine o'clock in the morning before I can see my mother again or speak to anyone on the stairs. My bed is like the shelf my toys are on, and I in my glass bottle put away like them, up out of reach.

And I don't like the clock either. It tells lies.

My mother says treats are like pennies which you save up in a money box. I think Time is something you save up too, and you spend it when visitors come. Then it's all gone till the next time.

Anchored into the armchair all these years later, I know this child from photographs: a skinny-legged creature, scrubbed clean, wearing a short frilly skirt, masses of ribbons on her ringlets, white ankle socks and shiny black shoes with a button on the side. She is timid and anxious at the same time. What I hadn't seen in her before was the determination as she tries to burst into life.

There are letters on my study desk, and I fetch them. They're from readers, from the outside world, from when I wrote books – and people wrote back to me. What I most want, more than anything else, is to get out of my glass bottle, to break into life again and become the capable person they wrote to. I want my body back, the one I lived in before with its strong spine, co-operative limbs – and working hands. I want to be spontaneous again.

The calculating nature of measuring pain has made me small, inward-looking, mean, frightened, withdrawn. It seems like a previous lifetime when I moved without thinking. Something must be done. Christmas is near and, as the shortest day of the year approaches, I stir in my chair and reach for the phone.

Chapter Six

❧

Finding Renzo

The hospital administrator is pleased to get my call. Yes, he says, he needs hospital visitors, people who will sit with patients, and he is short of help at the moment.

The idea had come from a friend:

'You need company,' she had said, 'and you'll be good at it.'

A few days later, questioning my motives for volunteering, the man at the hospital is relieved to hear they're limited.

'Do-gooders are a dangerous breed,' he growls from behind his overcrowded desk. 'You get people who think they're Florence Nightingale, and the next thing you know they're ordering nurses around and creating mayhem.'

Convinced I won't do this, he gives me an identity badge, and lets me begin. How long I spend on the ward is up to me: three to four hours, with a lunch-break in between, is about average.

My job is to do fetch and carry things for patients: to take a message; make a phone call; bring a sandwich; organise pen and paper. Especially, it is to sit and listen to people, to keep them company and spend the kind of time with them which nurses used to be able to do. Assigned a ward where there are twenty-four surgery and long-term-stay patients on the main floor and six people needing specialist care in side wards, I look forward to my first day. Listening to people is what I can do – and it's what I want, other people's stories instead of my own.

It's January, and after more than six months of incapacity, depression has been closing like sea fog round my armchair at home, threatening to cut me off altogether. The hospital soon becomes my way of being in the world.

Some patients are on the ward for many months. There's the window cleaner who has multiple broken bones from falling from the top floor of a house. He says the awful part was he had time to think how much it would hurt before he hit the ground.

As a journalist I've stepped over hundreds of door-steps, yet leaning over a stranger in a hospital bed seems wrong and, initially, I hang back, watch people's faces before approaching a man in a side ward.

'My name's Carol . . .' I begin.

His name is George, and he's one of life's victims,

born to a mother who was never without gin in her
handbag and a father who overused the strap. That
was fifty-six years ago. Things snowballed. He
developed drink and heavy smoking problems. Then
unemployment hit him. He's managed to knock off the
booze, but cigarettes are his company. By the time we
meet, George is bedridden, still smoking, and I'm his
only visitor. First of all he just talks. It takes two to three
months for him to ask me anything about myself and he
only listens to short, jokey answers.

The wonder is he survives at all. He's 32 stone – and
has just had a leg amputated above the knee. For a while
the stump won't heal, and he goes down to the operating
theatre twice again to have more of it removed.
Approaching the ward one day I have a vision of George
slowly disappearing before our eyes, inch by inch.
Instead, he recovers. He gets over first one infection,
then another, and is eventually discharged to a home by
the sea.

'Thanks for the visits,' he says before he goes. 'Do you
think I'll be needing my bucket and spade?'

Difficult though he's been, I miss George in the
following weeks: it's as if he took something of me with
him. There's such a lot of me missing by now that even
the words 'My name's Carol' have a hollow ring to them.
I'm all ears when it comes to other people's pain – but I
can't get a grip on my own.

I can't use a hairdrier any more, or iron. And since
buttons and zips are a problem too, I give up, and dress

like an invisible woman. I wear flat shoes so as not to fall over, floppy T-shirts and layers of clothes on top to fend off the cold.

In the house I once owned, the cats pretend I'm see-through and play 'Gosh, we didn't know there was anyone there' games with me. They do things like almost bump into me and then give outrageously fake impersonations of being shocked. Or, if I'm eating lunch with one of them nearby, she suddenly leaps stiff and four-pawed in the air when I reach for the salt. But I'm on to this lot by now and I don't let them rattle me.

At the surgery I don't let the doctor rattle me either. She wants me to see someone else, *another* physio-therapist, and she's insistent: 'I've seen her myself,' she tells me, 'and she's tremendous. You must go. You'll be better in no time.'

This is tricky. I won't be touched now. I can't afford to take another risk. Not yet. The friend who gave me Hannah got her address from his sister, who's a doctor. The physiotherapist I saw before her, who made me worse, came via another doctor. So I learn to lie at the surgery:

'I'm fine,' I say, picking up a Sick Certificate. 'Things are getting better. I'm sure it won't be long now.'

The doctor's not the only person I lie to. As the weeks and months go by, I become more secretive, seldom speaking unless I have to. Except for the hospital ward, I stay in the house. I stop going to public places, steering clear of theatres, cinemas, pubs, restaurants, parties and any crowded place where I might be bumped into, jostled or caught out by a sudden pain.

I still go and see a particular close friend, Sandy, who doesn't let the difference in me overwhelm her. If I'm unco-ordinated or start wincing, we pretend it's not happening and just carry on talking. If most of my food is left on the plate because I'm choking and my arms won't work, then that's how it is. No fuss.

There's a man friend too who isn't defeated by the downward shift in me.

'You're not the incapacity,' Peter says, urgently, after I've fallen foul of a few electric shocks and am sitting, grey-faced, nursing my arms, telling him to go away and leave me till the pain's gone.

'You're still the person you were before,' he insists. 'You've got an incapacity on top, that's all. You and the affliction are different. I don't care how many times you wince. You're still you.'

But am I? He's urging me to keep sight of myself as a strong woman when he doesn't know how gone from the world I am.

Something else I do at this time is enrol for night classes in Welsh, the language my mother never taught me. We're a strange assortment in the class. My stiff body and limited arm-use are no odder here than a Bosnian student's sudden appearance in our midst from finding a Welsh dictionary in a book-aid parcel. And there's a man who turns up to fall asleep each week – as if he couldn't do it without us.

With me, the words I heard as a child have lodged inside the ledges of my mind and now out they pop. Soon I have a quirky eloquence, as though I've dropped my fluent, polished English words for some nearer-to-home, hand-me-down Welsh ones. The night the electric shock strikes me here, I survive and go back the following week as if nothing had happened.

The hospital, patois Welsh: through the dark winter months, I retrieve a little of myself, of the woman I once was. Reading too. With the help of a book rest propped up on the table, I scan books – about the body mainly – trying to make sense of what's happened: more detective work, searching libraries for what's wrong with me, digging, cross-referencing, digging deeper again.

I learn it's not possible for a physiotherapist or osteopath to diagnose what's happening a lot of the time. This startles me. In my ignorance I imagined they could 'tell' things, like a doctor reads an X-ray result or blood test. But while some areas of the body are 'mapped' and easily recognised, others are not.

These are connective tissues, something I've not heard of before: large areas of tissue, also called fascia, which connect bones to muscles to form small tendons and linking parts all over the body. They don't show up on X-rays.

Books on how the body works also tell me it needs a variety of movements to be healthy. Too many fast 'tight' actions in a confined space are bad for it.

In the reading, I come across an article by broadcaster and columnist Allison Pearson describing her experience of something called RSI (Repetitive Strain Injury). The gist of the article is that RSI is still barely recognised by the medical profession. Yet tens of thousands of people get it, often from using computer keyboards, but also from other repetitive jobs in factories – and from playing in orchestras. When Pearson herself had RSI, the pain drove her home from the newspaper office where she worked. She describes how some of the other journalists who stuck it out are now permanently disabled.

A few weeks later, going along to meet a group for RSI sufferers organised by the National Union of Journalists, a reporter tells how he spent years recovering from the damage done to him by a chiropractor, his version of Hannah. Another man is back at work on a national newspaper, but a friend of his has committed suicide because of RSI. I remember the phone call from the man at the tennis club.

There isn't anyone in the room who got better quickly. Some will not get well at all. Most have tried five or six different kinds of treatment and many different practitioners before getting lucky. But what kind of condition is it? And do I have it anyway? Listening to what people say, I continue to trawl through library books, medical journals, newspapers and magazines.

Some of my reading during these winter months takes place by a log fire in Maidstone, Kent, where an aunt and uncle invite me to share hearth space at weekends. From friends of theirs comes the suggestion to see a Frenchman called Renzo Molinari. He's head of the European School of Osteopathy in Maidstone and a friend of a friend of my aunt's. I'm persuaded to see him because he'll be happy just to advise me. He won't touch me unless I want him to.

But the night before, I'm in a quandary. There's a problem with me seeing anyone now, not just fear of being physically hurt, but of being robbed of what I know. By this time, I'm sure my body's trying to tell me something. Unable to use words, it tugs at me, wanting my attention, and I'm beginning to take notice. When it says pavements are full of potholes, and to hang on tight to bannisters on the hospital stairways in case I come a cropper, I don't think it's forgotten how to walk, or what reality is. I think it's trying to remember something. I believe it's giving me a message – and I don't want Renzo Molinari, or anyone else, pouring scorn on this.

At the same time, I yearn for someone to help me. It's been more than six months on my own and I need assistance. But is Renzo the right person? Will he be another Hannah?
Some days I'm glad it's *my* life I'm taking risks with and nobody else's.

It's deep winter, and at our first meeting, Renzo, too, has the air of a detective, listening carefully to the story I tell him, hunting for clues. He is easy to talk to: still, alert, with a hint of charm or gallantry –

perhaps his Frenchness. Fortyish, slightly on the tall side, with dark eyes and hair, he has an air of thoughtfulness.

I give him factual information first: a list of the symptoms; when they began; how they developed; the X-rays I've had; the different people I've already seen and what they said was wrong with me; my time with Hannah, the traction headache and my trouble with swallowing. I describe the RSI group, some of the reading I've been doing, and show him the Allison Pearson article. I tell him about my enforced stillness in order to avoid pain, and he nods:

'Yes, I can see by your body.' In a flat, quiet voice, I say how afraid I am of the prospect of never getting better. I keep to myself the inner diving and feeling I don't any more fill out the space under my skin, say instead how I can't afford to have what little I can be sure of ridiculed. I tell him about my body's difficulty with imaginary potholes and the problem of describing any of this to anyone any more for fear of being thought mad. There, I've said it.

'No, no, you are not mad,' he says. He speaks English slowly, with a heavy French accent. 'It isn't — how do you say? — a piece? — ah, a figment — of your imagination. It's a sign of a problem with neck muscles.'

'Do you understand why I'm so afraid?' I ask, just before leaving. 'It's about trust. If you say you can help me, and then fail . . .' I don't say the rest.

On our third meeting, I manage to allow him to

examine me, to touch me enough to form an assessment of what he thinks is wrong. I breathe in and out at his request, lift an arm, move a wrist, bend a finger, as he feels along my spine, neck, arms, head.

'I can help you,' he says at last.

'Are you sure?'

'I wouldn't say it if I wasn't sure.'

'So what is wrong with me?'

He takes a deep breath. To begin with, he says there are a number of things wrong with me by this time resulting from what he calls a 'chain of injury'. He describes how sometimes a problem in the body can take years to reveal itself, especially if there's a long history of misuse. It will begin with a small injury, in an arm, say, which then begins to affect other neighbouring tissues and muscles as they try to 'help' the injured area cope. In other words, neighbouring parts of the body try and compensate for the injured party by propping it up and doing some of its work for it.

Renzo explains that the body is designed to do this, to be adaptive, and has many back-up facilities to cope if one part of it fails. Sometimes these adaptive measures work. Sometimes they don't, and instead of rescuing the injured limb, the rest of the arm becomes 'ill' too, and the shoulder along with it, from the effort of compensating.

In this way, the strain is passed on instead of being resolved and backs up, muscle by muscle, tendon by tendon, along the arm towards the spine. A domino effect. You eventually end up going to the doctor with a neck or a shoulder ache which began in a wrist or an elbow a year ago. By this time, there is a long chain of complicated injury to sort out mainly in the dark. It's in the tissue or fascia which connects muscles, as well as the muscles themselves.

Muscular tests can be done, but you still can't be certain which parts of the chain are weak links, which are stronger ones, and which links may 'give way' altogether if you try and work on them. So you move tentatively and it takes time. Here Renzo shrugs, as if explaining to me, tacitly, what went wrong with Hannah. She moved too fast.

He also explains how journalists and writers get these kind of injuries frequently because of the tense way they hunch forward and chase thoughts and ideas on to the screen or the page. He mimics this with his own body.

'See,' he says, 'the body comes forward, especially the neck . . . How do you say it in English? – when you stick out your neck and you catch something?'

He is looking for the phrase: 'You catch it in the neck.'

He acknowledges some tension is essential to creative work – and other kinds too – but says it has to be kept in balance. Perhaps he spots the guilty look on my face.

'So,' he demands, 'how many hours a day did you stick out your neck, and how fast did you chase the words?'

I don't tell him that sometimes it was the words chasing me, but my silence gives him his answer, and he goes on:

'There is no reason why you shouldn't work hard. Almost as hard as you like – almost. But you can only do this if you take care of the body. And then – I think the words in English are – if you take care of the body, the body will look after you.'

Chapter Seven

❦

How Now, Brown Cow?

That evening, a woman I've met at the RSI group comes round for a meal. Nothing complicated – it's the first time I've cooked for someone for a long time – and, to begin with, things are fine. We even laugh about taking ages between us to get the cork out of a bottle of wine. A fly on the wall would not have spotted either of us as incapacitated.

Then, like a mask slipping, I see it in her face, the cost of her effort. Large dark circles form round her eyes, mocking her brief freedom. She is crumpling. Her time is up, and now, swiftly, she must go home.

At the next session, I ask Renzo what he would do if I let him treat me. He explains he would do no 'adjustment'. He is not going to click my neck, or manipulate my body, at least not for a long time. He will start with cranial and 'inhibition' work to begin to relieve some of the tensions in the upper part of my torso to allow it to receive a better supply of blood and oxygen.

But, having got this far, I hold back. Suddenly I feel stampeded. It seems ridiculous, now, not to let him begin working on me. Yet I'm tormented by the memory of what I felt after Hannah.

Renzo's different though. He's listened carefully, given me time, and his description of how the body functions as an intelligent organism is reassuring. Some of the books and articles I've dug out take a similar point of view: that the body is hard-working, capable and obliging in its own right. Within its confines, it's a sociable organism with blood going round from place to place, calling here and there, nerves carrying messages back and forth, and muscles doing their best for their neighbours. This fits with my idea that my body's trying to tell me something.

Renzo describes how, when a part of the body is in trouble, other parts, not just the neighbouring ones, help out too. Veins, arteries and lungs provide ongoing as well as emergency support. The problem with workaholic writers is their habit of sitting hunched up and cross-legged so their lungs and veins can't function at their best.

My first lecture, and there'll be many more. I will learn that as well as being obliging and gregarious, the body is also forgiving – which is perhaps more than can be said for a mind like mine.

When I see him again, he's blunt:

'I cannot help you' he says, 'if you will not let me touch you. It is up to you.'

It is our fifth meeting and, except for a brief examination, we have only talked, I sitting on one chair, he on another. Sometimes standing up to show me something on one of the many large, coloured diagrams on the wall, or simply to walk around. My eyes have followed him. I have stayed put.

The dream goes like this:

I'd gone into the kitchen and there, standing large as life, was a full-size healthy golden-brown cow. She was plump and gorgeous, her smooth tawny hide shining with health.

I left the house, and when I returned, this creature had changed into a male 'cow'. Not a bull. The same cow as before – but, in some indefinable way, male instead of female. Now, instead of standing, it was lying on the floor in a pitiful condition. Its previously sleek skin was scuffed up, scabbed and peeling off. Rotting flesh was coming away in chunks with it. The animal was falling apart, dying. To my horror, it offered me a piece of its own flesh to eat. When I refused, it began to eat it up itself. The creature was devouring itself alive.

Around this time, eight months into the incapacity, I do two things. The first is to join Kew Gardens where I go to walk regularly, catching an overland train from North

London. It's early February. Kew is quiet and still and I'm not afraid of the Big Guns here. Although I'm exposed out in the open, and an easy target, there are large trees with their grey, brown and dappled trunks to shelter among. In time, a male golden pheasant comes to feed from my hand, and small birds too: blue tits, great tits and a robin.

The second thing I do is let Renzo Molinari treat me. A jolt soon follows. He tells me I should keep diary entries or a notebook of the pain in exact detail – time, duration, severity, place, activity when it occurred. All should be recorded.

'You do know I can barely write,' I say, with more than a tinge of sarcasm.

'Keep a record the best way you can,' he replies. 'You have to be patient.'

Patience! Who does he think is paying my bills? What does he think it feels like sitting day in, week out, month after month watching the world go by?

But we have a 'contract'. He will make me 80 per cent well within a year, and 90 per cent of my normal self by the end of eighteen months – *if* I learn to be patient.

So I write:

8.20 a.m. Tues. Sudden shooting pain in right arm. Right arm bad all day – stinging nettle and bruised sensations. Vice-like pains threatening.

Another entry:

6.20 p.m. Wed. Neck uncomfortable. Return of swallowing problem. Bad. Feel am choking. Also feel sick.

How much I manage to get down depends on my mood and how much arm-space I have. As well as the effort of it, there is the problem that I can't find a pattern in the 'evidence'. The entries accumulate daily without apparent reason or discernable clues.

8 p.m. Wed. Have to go to bed. Can't lift dictionary, can't do crossword, can't read. Lie still on back, looking at ceiling . . . Wish this weren't happening.

Treatment 28th March. Loaded trolley and carried shopping short distance. Debilitated by 'nerve' pain in right arm. Down bags.

Over about three months, between February and April, the pain notebook grows fat, taking up most of my arm-use. It becomes something in itself, and I don't like it – all that pain shut up in a book. I ask Renzo why I have to write things down in such detail and get the unobliging reply that it will become obvious in a little while – if only I will be patient.

Some days the notebook feels more important than I do. Me just a cypher for a pen and the notebook greedy. If I *am* on my way out, what an ignominious end, to disappear into a pain notebook. None of the laughter of me recorded there, nor the dancing on tabletops. It won't do. I begin to 'colour' my book:

Mon 25th. Pain back of neck and top back *left* shoulder (would have said without the notes always right shoulder that caused problems).

At night couldn't sleep, tried to be positive, counting sheep no good, thought of colours instead. RAINBOWS.

Think of seven colours, and seven shades of the desert in the Middle East . . . must have fitfully slept.

[Undated] The only thing to learn from these notes doesn't seem to help me: that memory is faulty, and I would say I was well when the day before I had been terrible, or vice versa. When this is over – oh, note the WHEN! – will I be free to move as before, or shall I be terribly different?

Oh blast, arms packed up.

[Undated] My body must be trying to make itself better. It's struggling.

Me writing in more things helping I think.

The *factual* bits of these entries I read back to Renzo each time we meet. Information for him, I think, to help him to make me better. He listens carefully, but rarely comments. When I ask a question – like why I should get a return of the electric shock treatment when I've barely moved my arm — his answer is direct, but doesn't seem to help:

'If you think about the position of your neck when the pain comes . . .'

But I don't remember where my neck is. I know what my arms were doing because that's where the pain is, but I can't watch myself all the time. I say this, that if I'm too careful, self-consciousness will do me in.

'You don't have to watch all the time,' he responds. 'When you get a bad pain, think about what you were doing with your neck and your spine, and not just with your arms.'

Living with a variety of pains, I have developed a personal vocabulary by this time, like a word-picture, for what is happening in my body. The heavy pain on top of my right shoulder I call the Black Dog because it feels like a heavy old Labrador draped round me. Words like 'vice', 'iron finger', 'travesty' and 'affliction' get used, as well as Big Guns. Iron Finger is the most personal. It's the feeling of being singled out for punishment: 'You will not work. You will not move. You will not drink coffee. You will not do anything unless I say so.'

'Insult' is a word I use too. It's from reading how insult and illness used to mean the same thing. The body's health was thought to be 'insulted' by disease, which is what I feel: shamed; demeaned. But what is my insult? Does it have a proper name? What is it that Renzo is treating me for exactly? I ask him.

'Inflammation of the connective tissues' is what he

says I have, the network of tissues, or fascia, which connects muscles and bones. He explains the problem like this:

'Nerves run through these tissues. The pain in your body is when inflammation causes the channels which the nerves travel through to be squeezed or restricted. That is when you get what you call an electric shock.'

But how did I get into this mess?

He says there are four main reasons or causes for it. The first is: I've suffered some injuries from the past I've kept quiet about. There's what he describes as a bad injury to my spine or neck, for example, which has made my neck a target. This doesn't make sense to me. Until now, I've never been to a hospital, or even inside a GP's surgery with a back or neck complaint. I would know if I had.

The second cause is simple. I'm prone to inflammation – and a change of diet will help. He suggests reducing coffee and cheese, no oranges, but grapefruit instead, no cooked tomatoes, raw is all right, not too much champagne . . . We both laugh.

The third problem is the one we've talked about: general overwork combined with bad typing posture. I've sat too long at a desk, hunched forward with my muscles tensed up. But there's also the problem of the old injuries I can remember nothing about. Renzo insists that muscles in the upper part of my body are defending injuries which I've put out of my mind. This is hard to believe. Surely I wouldn't forget being badly hurt?

The fourth, Renzo hesitates before explaining. There's an 'emotional component' in my condition, he says, some big emotion I'm holding on to and covering up. This irritates me. I've come to see an osteopath, not a psychotherapist.

He is quietly insistent:

'I'm telling you there's an emotional part to this only you can do something about. I can't. I can tell you what's in your body. Only you know what's in your life.'

The phrase 'what's in your life' takes the ground from under me, for what's in my life at the moment is frustration, pain and anxiety. How dare he talk about what's in my life. How could he possibly know what it feels like not to work, week after week, month after month, and to be in pain? At the next session I confront Renzo.

'Are you calling me neurotic?' I ask.

'You're not neurotic. Why do you think having emotions is neurotic? We all have emotions all the time.'

'But you're saying my emotions are making my body ill'.

He stops me: 'No. I'm saying this is a part of your problem. Your body is carrying a memory of something, some early physical trauma ·which you've defended yourself against. Your body has old injuries, and your mind is not telling me about these.

'You tell me you've never been injured. Go away and think. You're carrying bad injuries from the past. Your muscles and the tissues connecting your muscles have defended these injuries – and they're still doing it. Your body is out of its natural balance. That's why it's hurting. It's suffering for something in the past.'

Chapter Eight

❧

ONE HELL OF A GOD

Memory is a big place and if my body's suffering from something in the past, I can't find out what it is. But I recall something else. My father didn't like the sight of me with a pen or pencil in my hand or the sound of my voice either. In my father's church, God's voice was the only valid one and children's ways with words had, quickly, to be taken from them. Being an optimistic, talkative kind of child, I would keep on speaking up, as if by right, which is when the wholesale construction of a person called the Good Girl began.

It started when my mother, my father and myself lived in the flat in Sanderstead where my mother wrapped Time up in parcels for me and the clock told lies. We stayed in the house when I was between three and almost five years old.

Sanderstead was a nice place, a hilly area with a peaceful, rural feel to it. As well as the communal stairways which were my playing fields, there was a long lawned garden at the back where I also played. At the end of this garden there were mature trees which hid, in summer time, the big houses beyond.

After the war my father, who had been a flight engineer, left the RAF and we moved to Sanderstead to be near his mother in Purley. He was an only son and had married much against his mother's wishes. He had also gone to war against her pleas that he was too young – which he was. But the Luftwaffe's bombing of London had relieved his mother of one of her legs, and he promised her as she lay white as a sheet in a hospital bed that he would get them for that. Which he did.

He was one of the youngest men to volunteer, and those near him said he led a charmed life. Flying in Lancasters at night he twice came down over Germany and walked out over the French border both times, not a broken bone to be tended, barely a bruise on him. Unlike the targets beneath him in the dark, he seemed indestructible. Out over the channel with a bellyful of bombs, back again without them, out and back, out and back, trip after trip.

While the men around him were disappearing, already furled up into a long roll-call of the brave dead, my father was returning for operation after operation. Towards the end of the war, he landed a damaged Lancaster in a Lincolnshire airfield when the rest of the crew were badly injured. He saved their lives, although airmen's lives by that time had proved heavily expendable. As valuable for the war effort was the body of the plane itself.

When the odds against him coming back seemed impossible, the war ended, but not before he had taken part in the bombing of Dresden. It was the early hours of Valentine's Day when the mission was completed – my father's twenty-fourth birthday. He was one of 800 British Lancaster crews who had begun to demolish the city at midnight.

In all the paperwork that followed, there were com-mendations, rubber stamps and waxed seals which were eventually turned into a number of medals to be presented to my father by King George. Newspaper archives inform us the King was there at the Palace that day. My father was not. He was working in Civvy Street, trying to put the war behind him. For more than thirty years, he didn't speak of it again.

Although there was never a scratch on the outside of my father, the war was not over for him, and I began to be affected by this when I was about four. My father's mother, who lived near us, went to church, and my father too. My mother did not. Neither did I. She didn't believe small girls should have to – and my father and his mother were not pleased.

This was the time when I first remember hearing about God and His special interest in my behaviour. He had been invented, it seems, just to stop me from being naughty. Small girls were often naughty, my father informed me. They were made like that, and you couldn't always see it, this naughtiness, but it was there. And God, who had made all the world and the people and animals, didn't like it. It made him cross, and when God was cross, He told your father.

I mustn't think I could be naughty when Daddy wasn't looking because God was watching me all the time. He lived in the sky and could see everything I did. He could even see inside my head. He could see me under the blankets too *and* if I was playing with Teddy and when I was by myself. So I must do as Daddy says. I wasn't to talk to Mummy about God because she didn't understand Him the way Daddy did, so He was a secret between Daddy and me.

There were regular God talks after this about how naughty girls made bad things happen in the world, especially if they ever told lies, had bad thoughts – or made mistakes. A mistake was the same as doing it on purpose. So began a life where I was surveyed for any sign of error. And yet my father's idea of badness covered most of the ground a child would tread in a normal sort of day.

Tip-tapping down the stairs one morning, I was looking forward to there being lots of things in the day for me to see and count. Almost at the bottom, doing a twirl, my father raged out of the kitchen, and back to my bedroom I was sent. The rules were: I was to be obedient at all times; I was not to make a noise; not to get dirty; not to be a nuisance; not to skip in the house; not to slide on the bannisters; not to get in the way; not to answer back; not to run down the stairs and not to jump around.

But still, and still, my toe would tap. It was in me.

It was the 'bad thoughts' that were really hard to work out. They were to do with my body, which had been given to me by God. He had loaned it to me, so it wasn't really mine, and when I went to Heaven I would have to give it back to Him again. God had made my body, just like He had made all little girls and boys and I mustn't forget this, especially in places like the bath. Propped up by my elbows in the water, chin on chest, frown on forehead, I glared up and down myself looking for this badness God could see and I couldn't.

'Have you got something on your leg?' my mother asked.

I gave it to her to look at.

'Is it itching?'

I shook my head.

Later, when I cleaned my teeth, my head was full of pigeons from Trafalgar Square. Then I remembered God and looked round to see if He was watching me. I tried to make a picture of Him, but it was too hard. I knew He had lots of eyes and I also knew He talked to my father about me because of what happened when I was playing with my dolls.

Standing by the settee, I sat them in a straight line, telling them off as I went along: 'Now you sit there and behave yourself.' Sometimes my favourites, Jennifer and Priscilla, sat next to each other, and sometimes they sat one at one end and one at the other. Sometimes I changed them round a lot before I made up my mind, and got them where I wanted. This is when it happened.

'Have you been a naughty girl?'

His voice, as big as the house, makes me jump – my father come to get me. And, suddenly, everything in the room changes size. My father is so big I can't see the top of him, and the settee is big now and everything is growing so much bigger than me. The ceiling of the room has gone up into the sky . . . and I am getting smaller.

As my father leads me off by the hand, I'm terrified I will disappear.

The interrogation of a four-year-old is a dreadful affair.

'Have you been a naughty girl?'

'You have, haven't you?'

'What have you done?'

I am not allowed to say nothing. That's cheeky.

Another afternoon at a dolls' tea-party, I'm playing mummy again. There's real milk and sugar, and the cups and saucers from the dolls' house are on the table: I'm carefully pouring milk into a cup. Then it's there, as big as the fat end of a pencil, a drop spilled on the table; round, white. And he's there too, my father, and I'm trapped: him on one side of me; the wrong drop on the other, and I am led away by the hand. Playing mummy to my dolls one minute, I am all of a rag doll myself the next.

My lies begin then. Taken off for another stern talk, this is where I give myself away, for I'm so confused, I confess to anything. Yes, I am naughty and yes, I have to be punished. My father so often finds me out, catching me unawares so that I jump, and this means I must be guilty. So . . .

Yes I spilled the milk.

And what else have I done he demands.

I try to think.

Because the room gets angry with me and grows so big it frightens me, I know I must have done something really bad. But I can't remember what it is, and there's a big bird banging its wings inside my chest and it wants to get out. The more my father asks me things, the more my words get jumbled in my head and they want to fly out with the bird, but I don't want them to go away. I want to keep them.

My father's height – six feet – adds to his power over me. He seems like God up in the sky, and my own shrinking at the sound of his voice makes him taller. That's the trouble with naughty girls. One spilled drop of milk and the world changes: things start to move, to grow big and frightening, and the things you like disappear.

So this is the beginning of my terror: the bird trying to get out of my body; the room changing size; me getting smaller; my words, the ones I like the sound of and practise saying slowly like my mother, flying away. I'm terrified there will be no girl left. She'll be all gone.

The punishment for all this mayhem is a hiding, and

then to be left afterwards by yourself with no pencils, toys or books. This is the worst bit.

Wandering around by myself, looking at things in the room, I try to find something which belongs to a child. I long for a book, a coloured crayon, a doll that I can be friends with. There is nothing here.

The place where this happens, where I am locked in, is my parents' bedroom, next to the living room, and it's carpeted and furnished. Yet I think this room is bare: bare wooden boards on the floor; nothing on the walls; no furniture except an old wooden kitchen table. Sounds, colours and toys have vanished and a place friendly to children has disappeared.

I come to know two worlds. One has dolls, furniture, people, colours, sounds and normal shapes. Then, a tilt, and everything I think is safe is thrown into a different shape and size. I don't know how to get the safe things back and make them all right again.

The first bit of resistance I remember having in the battle between my father, his Old Testament version of God and myself was a piece of innocence. It came from being too young to understand something.

At the age of four I hadn't yet grasped the idea of things happening at the same time in different places. 'Simultaneous' was a concept I didn't know. I thought things happened, like numbers, one after the other.

So however many times my father said God watched me every single minute, I knew this couldn't be true because He had to watch other people and animals too. That was His job, to watch people, and to do that He had to go to other people's houses sometimes – which meant He couldn't be in ours at the same time.

If you're trying to control a child you have to know her mind. She can nod 'yes' as many times as you demand, and indeed she has been listening, but if her mind is free of the idea 'simultaneous', you can't tie her up in knots with it.

My second line of resistance was a resilient and subversive nature behind my good girl exterior. I was often cheerful when God and my father were out and I practised being a child of my own. While the good girl had to walk slowly, be quiet, smile nicely and never be rude, I stamped about the garden thumping my feet. I pulled faces and smacked bushes as well. Indoors, too, I deliberately did things I wasn't supposed to. I poked my tongue out at the mirror, smacked my dolls, jumped up and down and said things out loud just to see how big the sound was.

Sitting on the high, wooden-seated Victorian lavatory one day, I was swinging my legs slowly and trying to knock the back of my shoes against the bowl to see how loud *that* was. Pee finished, I was lolling lazily in a dream. Daddy was at work, Mummy in the sitting room, and God? Down from the seat I jumped, and then a quick turn round to stare down the U-bend. What a relief. No, God wasn't there. It must have been one of those times when He was watching someone else. I didn't say anything to my father about God's absences. I kept this to myself for the treasure it was.

When my father and God were away, my third form of escape was my talks with the rest of the street – and the world at large. I was a strong believer in communication skills and whether on walks with my mother or at home, I chatted to people: tram conductors; shopkeepers; neighbours; cats; dogs; coalmen; postmen; milkmen and widowers with bars of chocolate. A glimpse of a smile on a grown-up's face and I said hello. A friendly question about what I had been up to that day always got a long reply. I didn't leave anything out. I was talkative through the garden fence, on the tram and anywhere outside the house.

Using words of my own, practising them, rolling them round my tongue, hearing the sounds they made, and seeing the effect, I was seldom happier than when telling the neighbours all about myself. My mother seemed to approve of this, and the fact that she herself never talked about God, and wasn't very interested in Him, led me to feeling bold enough on occasion to try to get my father to yield a little.

Although I was afraid when he put on his strict voice and grew high as a church, I could not believe he wasn't on my side. Sitting on the table during the God talks I would sometimes try and persuade him. Maybe I could be allowed just a tiny bit of naughtiness and it wouldn't matter if I tripped over, hopped down the stairs or spilled some milk.

At my cheerful and beguiling best, I came up with an idea: maybe I could be naughty *sometimes* and maybe we don't have to tell God about it. This said looking round over my shoulder to see if I could spot Him. Forefinger and thumb held in the air on top of each other, I made a space between the two so they were almost touching. This is how much – and how little – time I wanted to be naughty for. But my father was not persuaded or convinced. A good girl is what I had to be – at all times.

What he couldn't stop me doing was growing. Neighbours said it to me lots: 'My, what a big girl you're getting to be', and I twirled round so they could see the bigness, stretched my arms up and stood on tiptoe. Eating up all my food made me bigger and I grew when I was asleep as well.

I'm quiet with Renzo the next few weeks. In the pact between us he has said he will tend my body while I take care of my life and I'm sticking to that. But the word 'childhood' hasn't been mentioned between us, and this is what I'm dealing with: a child's resistance to two giants, and her attempts to grow herself despite them.

They had both terrified me, yet one of them, my father, I also loved, and I turned myself head over heels and almost inside out to get him to love me back.

My father smiled when he was happy and he made me laugh by pulling silly faces. He did magic tricks with a ping-pong ball, which he swallowed or made disappear behind his back, and played catching the ball games with me in the garden.

I was to spend years trying to win my father. I turned somersaults, cartwheels, did headstands and hand-stands and tried every wishing-to-please, singing-and-dancing, busking-to-the-crowds trick I could think of to win his heart.

When this failed, I must also have begun the process of trying to save the life I was determinedly growing behind his back. I began to put away something of my own to feed on, to stow away in an invisible larder you have inside yourself for a certain kind of hunger. My larder, or den, was a secret and it was mine and it was a place where God and my father couldn't get to. God, who could see through bedclothes and buildings wasn't clever enough to find it because I hid things there when He wasn't looking.

A saving-up kind of child, I stored words, thoughts, parcels of Time, resistance, secrets, pictures, and I counted things too, inside my head: things I'd seen in the world outside, my eyes like a camera.

In years to come, what I hid in my den *would* save my life, but what I wasn't to know was that as I grew, and as my den grew with my secret resistance in it, so did my father's God in me.

Chapter Nine

❧

THE GIRL IN THE TRUNK

My father's refusal to accept my life, to love it, was known to me by the age of five and I understood it as his wish to kill me. Although death didn't mean the same to me as it does now, for I believed you could die and still wake up again in the morning.

My sense of being 'killed' came about because acceptance – love – was the centre of my child's world and I didn't exist without it. When my father grew tall as a church and I grew smaller and smaller, I was in thrall to the terror of being 'all gone'.

Something else came from my father, the feeling of being, always, too late. Too late was one of his ways of scolding me. If I asked him to repeat something because I wasn't listening or didn't understand, he would say: 'It's too late now. You've had your chance.' This could happen if I wasn't ready when he promised to take me out. Then he would go out without me and I would watch from the window as he disappeared down the road, crying because I'd been left behind.

In the days when she wasn't ill, the opening notes of *Listen with Mother* sent me to my mother's lap — my harbour — where life was warm, safe, intimate. Somewhere in these lap times I had fallen in love with being alive, with shapes, colours, textures and the voice coming out of the radio.

I'm hiding from Renzo. I don't want him interfering in my inner world. My emotions are my business, he has said, but does he know anything about them? Has he any idea of the weight of my, or anyone else's, past?

'What good will any of this sitting still and being patient do?' I ask him. 'I want to work. Other people work. You do. I just want to get back to work.'

'Yes,' he says. 'I know. And you will. But the problem is . . .' He explains again about the large amount of muscular tension in my body.

'The tension in the muscles of your right shoulder is holding your right shoulder forward in an unnatural position. One of your ribs is not relaxing when you breathe out, so it is permanently "proud". The muscles and fascia in your thorax are taut like a band of steel. You have deep muscle tension, and superficial muscle tension too. All the upper part of your body is in a defensive position, as if you are protecting yourself.

'Now, let me finish,' he says as I go to interrupt. 'So what I've learnt from your body is that you defend yourself against pain to such a big extent that your body is suffering. If my shoulders were suffering what yours are suffering I wouldn't be able to do my job or live my life. I can't help you if you won't help yourself. I don't know your past injuries. Only you can know them.'

Stung, sometimes, by the thought that my incapacity, my life, is my fault, I'm struck by Renzo's comparative ease. Time seems to stretch for him. In the waiting room, with students, with staff, he is attentive, courteous and unhurried. I, on the other hand, am torn. Part of me accepts my luck in finding Renzo. I also find him difficult.

The link between mind and body I half understand. If I were well, perhaps all of me could accept it. The part that's struggling is something to do with the imbalance between Renzo and me. He's the person standing on his feet, earning a living, leading a full life. I'm the one lying down, everything on the line. What right does he have to put me through more and where might it lead? Will I be safe in his hands?

He is uncompromising: 'I can work on the muscles. Only you can work on the mind. Bodies and minds are not separate. If your mind or heart is hurt, then that hurt shows in your body. I can help to release physical tensions. You have to take care of the emotions. That's what I'm saying. You don't have to tell me anything about them. You just have to know them yourself and your body will improve.'

One day I ask him about exercise. I've started doing

some slow, cautious yoga again, but it's difficult to judge how much pain is acceptable. Should I stop if a movement hurts just a little bit or should I carry on through the pain? How much should I do each day? Are there other exercises that would help?

'You are trying too hard, you know,' he says. 'You are creating tension from trying. If you try too hard you make yourself more tense. But –' he pauses – 'you are slowly improving.'

Tears start to pour down my face as I hear the magic words: 'slowly improving'. Improvement. There's improvement!

'How much improvement?' I ask, hurriedly wiping my face.

'Enough,' is the reply.

There is slight easing in the muscular tension in my body, enough to tell him we are on the way and will get there.

'Now, I will say it to you again, you will be well. It will take more time. You will need more patience. This is the beginning of a journey upwards. But,' he warns, 'you will slow things down if you don't relax and accept that the body needs time to heal itself.'

The warning flies by me at first, for I don't know where to put myself for joy. I want to dance, skip, fling my arms in the air. And then I realise something: I have hunched up my shoulders with excitement and I'm not breathing. My arms, neck, head, back are rigid; feet, ankles, knees too. For an instant, it's all there, the evidence. Locked muscles; taut, fixed posture; a frozen frame. For the first time, I know what he means about the tension because, for the first time, I feel it.

Slowly I allow myself to breathe properly and let my shoulders down again, unstick my feet from where they've been clamped to the floor, and release the muscles in my neck. Is this what I've been doing all these years, especially with work, tensing all of my body up as I get an idea? Then, not letting myself breathe or relax till I've tracked it down, flung it up in the air, shaken it around, jumped up and down on it and finally flattened it into submission.

Sometimes you wait so long for something to happen, you don't recognise it when it does. Sitting at home, I've been seeing repeated images for weeks before at last I take notice of what's showing on my inner screen.

The girl is around four and a half. She is a happy skipping kind of child and is laughing as she steps – no, almost dances – into an open-lidded trunk placed behind a bedroom door. The 'video' of this goes back and forth, like a fast 're-wind, then play' sequence many times before it slows down and eventually plays at normal speed.

The brown-eyed, dark-haired girl who stepped or danced into this trunk was laughing. The trunk itself was half metal, half wood, with a heavy, round, combination lock. When open, this lock dropped down, hanging loose on its brass hinge. Closed, you clipped its round face up against the body of the chest into a dial. You locked it with a twist of the metal top in the dial and you had to know the right number of twists to make it spring open again. Covered with a tablecloth, the girl roaming around her parents' bedroom in the Sanderstead flat took no notice of it.

The day the girl danced into the trunk, or box as she called it, she was playing a game of hide and seek with her mother and father. It was one of those happy times when they all played together as a family. Her daddy was at home and her mother was 'it'. The girl and her father ran into the other room, the parents' bedroom. They looked around:

'Quick' he said, pulling off the table-cloth and opening the trunk lid, 'in here.'

In she jumped.

Putting back the cloth, the clasp, sticking out at the side, was a giveaway untidiness. Quickly he closed it.

As the box lid was shut, total blackness came on top of her. Then a click, a lock, and everything was gone: colour, sound, life. She couldn't see herself, no arms, no legs. And suddenly she knew. She had been waiting for it: her father had killed her at last. Too late had already happened.

Fifteen years after this incident, when the girl was nineteen, her mother told her: 'We couldn't get the trunk open again. The lock had stuck. We had to get a neighbour to prise it open. When we got you out, you were unconscious, but breathing. We decided to put you to bed and see how you were in the morning.'

In the morning, the girl woke up, as usual, seemingly unhurt. Her parents decided not to call the doctor and to forget the incident. They believed if a child didn't say anything, there was nothing wrong. It wasn't mentioned again, and they soon forgot it. The episode was buried so completely that when the child mentioned it in her thirties, when debilitating claustrophobia had reared its ugly head in her life, the parents claimed it had never happened at all.

Sometimes, in carefree or happy times, I am rid of this claustrophobia, but it comes back over the years. In a house in Hertfordshire one night, watching friends double lock all doors and windows and put security keys in safe places, panic begins and I spend the small hours in a chair looking at the stars, only feeling safe if I can see them.

Gradually, any enclosed space – the back seat of a car, a windowless committee room, one of the new sealed main line trains – anywhere where someone else has charge of opening or closing the doors, of keeping the keys, is difficult. Struggling with it, failure is what it seems to represent: a self-imposed handicap; lack of courage.

In Sanderstead, sitting up in the box, I began to travel at great speed. I started moving down a long slide in a tunnel. On and on it went in the dark, faster and faster, and I was frightened. I didn't believe I could sit up and go that fast without falling over and I felt I was losing my breath. Then, I wasn't in a tunnel any more. I was flying. I had flown out of the tunnel into the sky and now I was floating and now it wasn't dark. Stars. Millions of them, me in the middle.

But I wasn't a child any more. I wasn't a body. I don't know what I was: a cell perhaps, or a small single eye in all the starlight. I was out of the box, though, out of the nothingness and the place where I couldn't see myself or know the world.

And I could fly.

The trunk was the beginning of two skies for me. I already lived a life of two worlds, the friendly one with dolls and colours in it, and the frightening one where things tilted away from me. With the trunk, there arrived in my life one world where the sky was outside my head and the other where it was inside.

But can a child get out of a box?

Chapter Ten

❧

Auditioning for Fathers

I was removed from this first of many 'deaths' by my mother taking us off to Wales. We went to a small mining village in Carmarthenshire, where my Welsh grandparents lived, leaving my father behind in Surrey. Whether it was his attitude towards her, or me, or both of us which pushed her over the edge, I don't know, but she'd had one nervous breakdown and wasn't about to volunteer for another.

The first of many separations, it lasted a number of months. My father's mother, Nellie, was said to be partly to blame. Living near us in Sanderstead, she didn't like my mother. On my visits to see her, when we rang the bell and heard Nellie's slow, heavy footsteps coming down the hallway, I was left on the doorstep and my mother went away. She sat in a cafe or, if it was fine, walked around till my visiting time was finished.

But you had to be extra nice to Nellie. She had a wooden leg from the war.

Taking me aside before we set off for Paddington Station on our journey to Wales, my father's departing-from-London God talk went like this:

'God will still be able to see you in Wales, and if you do anything naughty while you're there, he'll tell me about it. Now, what are you to be? That's right. A good girl at all times.'

Well, that lasted as far as Slough. Oh, the excitement of the train, and the different people, and the chugging noise of the engine. Lulled by the underneath rhythm of dozens of wheels, the rhyme of them, the movement, the sound, the swaying carriage, the fields moving by my eyes, the houses, the cows, I thought trains were the best thing in my life so far.

My grandparents, Harry and Bessie, lived in a house with lots of people – my two youngest uncles, who were teenage boys, and Derek, a grandchild like me, and nine months younger. There was plenty of activity: children playing in the street; running footsteps from games; shouts; people's voices; murmurings, even at night, through the windows and walls.

The row of red-brick council houses was on a hill with a view of the sea only a few miles off and the black mountains in the distance. My mother went to work as a night nursing auxiliary and my grandparents looked after me while she slept in the day.

The child of my mother's middle sister, Derek had

been brought up by Harry and Bessie from when he was less than a year old. The house where our grandparents lived was his home and he called them Mum and Dad. I had a mother with me, but . . .

Straight to it I went, quarrelling with my cousin over our smiling, blue-eyed, story-telling grandfather.

Me: 'He's my daddy too.'

Derek: 'You've already got a daddy in England. He's mine.' Push, shove.

Me: 'But he's mine, so there.' A push back.

Derek: 'Yours is in England. You can't have mine.' Another push.

Me: 'Nana, tell him he's my daddy too.' Sob, wail.

An arrangement was reached. Yes, I did already have a daddy in England, and he was Daddy Lee, but for the time I was in Wales, I could have shares in Derek's daddy, and he would be called Daddy Williams. And yes, he was my daddy too.

So there we were, the three of us. And there was Harry, a loved and happy man, a small child on either hand both watching him like hawks for signs of favouritism. Harry dealt his favours well and, out on our walks, I was content with the Godless shape of the skies over Wales.

Harry's way with children was known in the village. Retired early from coal-mining due to pneumoconiosis, he spent time in the garden. Making mounds and trenches for potatoes and beans, there was often a child with him, trailing doll, shawl, tractor, or asleep under the hedge.

Bessie was different. Coming from a well-to-do family, she didn't like cleaning, cooking or anything in the house – except playing her beloved piano. Training to be a concert pianist before she married, seven children were a shock to her and sitting at the piano was where she was happiest.

But we were soon to leave Wales. In the next five years I was moved many times as my father changed jobs and continents trying to find a new beginning, a way of making things happy for us all. Travelling ahead of us to try out a new job, it was often months before my mother and I joined him. Without the security of a permanent daddy, I searched for a substitute when he was away, someone to believe in me and make my life safe.

Sometimes I went about this by advertising myself. So a man who smiled at my mother and me in a bus queue might get a big smile back from me followed by a detailed description of my life: my likes and dislikes; details of my travel and sleeping arrangements at the time; what I liked best to eat; character reports on some of the people important to me – and their culinary, marital and domestic details too. This was to show what a full and interesting life I led and how fatherhood of such a girl would be a rich and rewarding undertaking not to be missed. Shops, trains, pavements, doorsteps were all possible venues for me recommending myself in this way.

On a train once with my mother, squashed into a

compartment with six men in posh suits, I brought shame upon her with the following:

'I've got two daddies,' I declared. 'One lives in Wales and he's white, and he's Derek's daddy too, and the other one . . .'

Sometimes, though, I did things the other way round and expected likely fathers to prove themselves to me. On-the-spot auditions were conducted, vicars being especially vulnerable to my scrutiny. Knowing as I did the secret about God not watching *all* the time, I was on the lookout to test how many vicars were up to scratch. If fatherhood was on my mind that day, people like uncles, postmen and neighbours also had to watch out.

Before we left Wales, the father problem flared up again between Derek and me with the upsetting business of my being sent to sleep at my cousins' for my last weeks there. The house we all lived in at number 77 was too full, and only a few doors away Harry's sister lived with her three daughters at number 85 . The youngest girl, who was eleven, was sleeping in a big bed on her own, leaving room for another body.

There was no consultation of course. Grown-ups never think of things like a bit of warning or even a chat before a child has her pyjamas packed and is taken off down the street. And as well as leaving my mother's bed, the new arrangements meant Derek had the place we called 77 to himself at night. He was the only child there and he might steal Harry's heart while I was sleeping out. Sometimes he gave me an 'I've got more than you' smile when I was led away. I wanted to kick him. I was afraid that by the morning Harry wouldn't love me any more.

Trouble with my aunt didn't help my feeling of being left out. My mother's youngest sister was jealous of us both and she teased me a lot. I wasn't allowed to be cross with grown-ups, so I put up with her pulling my ringlets, tweaking my ribbons and putting on a silly voice. One day, I could take no more. Turning to her, I scrunched up my face as hard as I could and said:

'Oh you blinking . . .'

It was the biggest swear word I could think of at the time, and pre-dated by four or five years the children's swear-words-you-can't-get-a-hiding-for rhyme which I learnt on another visit to Wales:

The butcher threw the bloody knife
over the damn wall
it landed on the blinking stars
and ended up in hell.

So there. Smack me for that if you can.

While my mother and I were living in Wales, my English father had rejoined the RAF and gone to Suez. He had been writing to my mother and sending pictures of himself. He wanted us to go and stay with him and my mother had to decide. Should we stay in Wales with Nana, Daddy Williams and Derek, or should we go to Egypt? She asked her father.

'It's up to you,' he said.

After four months of being in Wales, of working nights and living in her parents' home, my mother made up her mind. We would live with Daddy Lee again and would be going on a boat to see him in this strange, hot country called Egypt.

Harry presented the news as very exciting. He huffed and puffed himself up into telling such amazing stories about hot countries that I couldn't wait to leave. I was halfway out the door by the time he had finished exclaiming what a lucky girl I was. Oh, so lucky. And while I was off seeing big ships, bigger than houses, and waves in the sea, and dolphins in the water, and ladies in veils, and sunshine all day long, and buckets and spades, and the colours of dancing girls' swirling skirts, Derek would have to stay behind in Wales. Poor Derek.

But before the journey back to Paddington to pack some clothes for Egypt, on the morning we were leaving, I stole something. It was something I'd been warned not to touch and couldn't put back. An irreparable crime and a memory – my first – of not being able to make things right again.

A dab of perfume is what I took. My cousin's. The bottle, like the rest of the ornaments on her dressing table, was out of bounds to me. But on that last day, the pressure of leaving Wales was too much and I cracked. All the way to London I stank of guilt and lily of the valley and expected to be arrested on arrival and put in prison.

Indeed, we did go on a boat to Egypt just a few days later, shortly after my fifth birthday. But there was a disappointment before we left England, a cloud on my carefree, brightly coloured, bucket-and-spade skyline. It came as we journeyed to Tilbury docks. My mother and I had the compartment to ourselves, with plenty of space for wriggling around and chatting, but she wasn't talking. Concerned about whether she had made the right choice in taking us away, she was pensive now that we were leaving.

Not me. Feeling my toes curling in my shoes with excitement – going on a boat for the first time, and such a big one, bigger than lots of houses – I had an idea. If the boat was that big, and Egypt was that far away, miles and miles, and much further than Wales, then maybe . . .

I felt sure of the answer by the time I asked the question. Big and clever though God was, He wouldn't be able to get to Egypt. I wouldn't have to be worried about Him any more. I was going to be rid of the Chief Spymaster, the watching figure who pulled at my mind and clouded my days.

'Will God be able to see me in Egypt?' I asked my mother.

'Of course,' she replied in a shushing tone of voice. Oh blinking, blinking, blinking . . .

Chapter Eleven

❧

EGYPT

The first problem with our time in Egypt was the journey. The boat we were travelling in, a troop ship called the *Charlton Star*, had seen heavy service and, halfway to Suez, started to leak.

Being five, sitting on the top bunk of the cabin eating dried biscuits while paddling my feet in sea water didn't especially trouble me. I was, in any case, receiving supplementary rations. I had taken up with the ship's chaplain and was being fed well-polished apples straight from the clerical pocket. Regaled with detailed accounts of His Maker's habits: from watching birds, animals, grown-ups – and children too – to His long chats with fathers; he said he had never known a five-year-old who talked quite so much about God.

For my mother, however, the crossing to Suez was forewarning, perhaps, of how unwise she may have been to take us away from the safety of Wales. Keeping me close by, her fear made me anxious too. Something was wrong.

In Egypt itself, some awful things happened. It was the beginning, for me, of *knowing* what the bad inside me was, of discovering my ability to 'kill' or lose people, and outside a war was brewing – a crisis in Suez. There was gunfire in the streets and my father had been sent away.

Originally stationed in Fayid, an RAF base twenty-five miles north of Suez, he was dispatched at short notice to fly in and out of Nairobi. For most of the ten months we lived in Egypt, that's where he was – flying over Libya, Ethiopia, the Sudan. His job was important. The British Government wanted aerial pictures of the Middle East and the Saharan region of Africa. Mapping thousands of square miles, RAF planes flew back and forth, grid by grid, cameras recording as they went, my father with them. So he wasn't there to protect us when, soon after we arrived, a nightmare happened in the middle of the night in the flat upstairs.

A woman was attacked. The sound of this, of crashing furniture, broken glass and someone being chased, carried through the open French windows. Woken by the sound of men shouting and a woman's screams, I ran from bed to where my mother was standing outside on the small front balcony shouting for the men to stop. Coming out on to the balcony above us, two of them, just feet above our heads, made as if to jump down. Threatening my mother, they told her to mind her own business or she would be next. We ran indoors, shut the French windows, front and back, then the shutters and the heavy metal bolts on top.

Standing in the dark in the living room, in the middle of the floor, my mother trembling, I clung on to her. But she wouldn't say anything and she seemed to be angry, telling me to go back to bed, but I wouldn't let go.

I could feel her going from me again, like she did in Sanderstead, withdrawing. I knew this mustn't happen in Egypt: it was a new country to me and I didn't know my way. So, hanging on tightly, I made pictures in my head of nice things. I thought about Nana and Daddy Williams and the safety of Wales. Then a wrong thing happened. I couldn't remember if I knew my grand-parents properly, if they were real, or if they were in my imagination. Did I know them, or had I made them up? Were they alive or had I killed them?

I was in a land I didn't know, my mother wasn't nice to me, and I didn't carry my grandparents inside my head any more. It would plague me years later – where people went to when I left them.

The rest of my stay in Egypt was marked by this, by disturbed nights when, getting up, I stood under the fan in the living-room ceiling, its gently swishing wooden blades and light air soothing me. By day I was moody.

The building we lived in was a six-storey concrete block with a flat roof at the top. The apartments had a small balcony at the front and a large one, running the width of the main bedroom, at the back. There was only one fan, the one in the living room, and with temperatures high inside and out, I was often thirsty.

Drinking water for the day arrived in the morning – a giant, oblong ice cube in a sack. The man who carried it on his back put it in a small metal cylinder in the kitchen. By evening it was always gone.

Outside in the day, sometimes it was calm in our street: murmuring voices; people walking slowly in the heat; and, through the heat haze, the vivid colours, scents and blue skies Harry had talked of. But then, shouting in the distance, and a swift change. The sound of guns, far away at first, then shooting, near now, and, more frightening by far, the sound of dozens – perhaps hundreds – of pairs of bare feet slapping hard on pavements.

If we were in a cafe when this happened we had to go home again quickly. It meant the mob were out with their warning cries of 'British out, British out.' The smell of danger strong, I blamed the camels; took against them, thinking they were random devourers of small girls. I shrank back from their lurching gait, haughty heads and ever-smacking lips. Or else, if I thought I was at a safe distance, I glared at them. I scratched and frowned a lot: prickly heat, insect bites, chafing clothes, damp hair, thirst and fed-upness.

Starting school in Egypt wasn't like the story books where your mother walked you to the school gates and you played games with other children. In Suez, you were

taken, by yourself, in a big army truck with a canvas
cover over it making it dark inside. Early in the morning,
you waited for the noise of the truck rattling round the
corner into your street. Then you went downstairs and
were lifted quickly by soldiers through the tent flaps at
the back of the truck into the gloom. You were handed
further back then, where it was even darker, and tucked
down to make sure you were safe. Journeying in this
way, you couldn't read your book or see where you were
going.

School was in an army camp, surrounded by a high
wire fence with soldiers marching round it with guns.
The teacher made us drink a bottle of goat's milk with
lumps in it and you weren't allowed not to. The milk was
warm and made you feel sick. You weren't allowed to
play outside either and I longed to get home again.

In the flat, there was company by this time – another
Forces wife and her two children. The biggest, Anne,
was almost a year younger than me, and a baby, Denise,
was nine months old. She became Chief Assistant in a
game Anne and I played when the boiling heat,
itchiness, bites and the angry patches on our bodies and
inside our heads finally got to us one morning. Denise
had a pot in the bathroom, and that is what gave us the
idea: we would potty bomb the flat downstairs.

I can't remember if we used the baby's Number
Twos, or whether we borrowed her pot to produce
original ones of our own. Anyway, whether first-hand
material or stolen from the baby, Anne and myself crept

on to the back balcony, and upended the potty's contents on to the verandah below: 'There, take that all you grown-ups. If you think you can go about your lives while small girls are fed up and put upon, and hot and sticky and scratching, well small girls will show you a thing or two. Take that.'

The poor man downstairs, who had done us no harm, must have wondered what had hit him – and why. But we quickly got caught. The game was too naughty and, after a couple of days, we set about producing our own comeuppance. Giggling in a loud, false way, we did exaggerated shuffling noises. The timing of the attacks was a give-away too, always happening first thing in the morning when our mothers were busy having their cups of tea. This was our way of pointing the finger at ourselves and saying: 'It's us. It's us. We're the ones.'

So it only rained Number Twos in that part of the world for a few days before the man downstairs was on to us.

I can't remember if it was Anne or me who thought up this piece of revenge. On the one hand, I think it must have been me because I was older. On the other, I think it must have been Anne. Given my reined-in, uptight, 'thou shalt not' upbringing, I could hardly be credited with it. How could a girl watched by God for any naughty thoughts plan this?

In the moves we made, leaving Suez was the first when I knew it was my fault. I believed I had the power to make us leave, that my having bad thoughts about a place was the reason it got left behind – and was sad without me. In my world of children's stories, objects had feelings too: toys; dolls; houses; chairs. Had I tried to make things better and nice for them? Or had I been a nasty, bad-tempered girl and not given things a chance?

My life in Egypt brought the conscious beginning, with guilt, of grief, anger, and my power to 'kill' places and people I loved. As my eyes devoured the world, and God with all his eyes watched me, I had the notion that people and places were dead if I couldn't see them. Watched as I was by this powerful God, I believed there was something crucial to life – and death – in my own gaze, too.

For there were aspects of Egypt I liked, which I was sorry to say goodbye to: the fan which comforted me in the night; the days we went to the beach; waving at soldiers and sailors in their deckfuls as their ships moved slowly along the canal. Standing on the side with my mother, ships so close you could see the smiles on the sailors' faces when they waved back, the world seemed a big, friendly place.

Within the year we left Suez. With mobs on the street attacking buildings now, and Anne, Denise and their mother already gone, my father came to fetch us. The first I knew of us leaving was being woken in the middle of the night and told we were going away.

'Will we be coming back?' I wanted to know.

Never understanding how to respond, over the years, to this – and many other – urgent questions of mine, my parents had a 'real' crisis to deal with. Already, a street-roaming gang had spotted our luggage downstairs in the lobby. Warning they might be back, the landlord urged us to leave without delay. They had, in any case, taken our baggage. All our possessions were gone.

Upstairs, I was trying to cope with the sudden loss of my home, of the things we did here – and their loss of me:

'I'll be sad when you go,' Harry had said, making a sad face, 'and the birds and trees will cry too.'

I needed time. I wasn't ready. There were too many wrong, frightening things in Egypt which I wanted to put right before I left: an army of red crabs once, near the sea, threatening to cut me off from the shore; grimacing camels; feet running on pavements; the hot building; this too-high room. I wanted to make things better.

Soon I wouldn't be able to see this room any more. It would vanish from my eyes and I would have killed it. I wanted to store it in my head where, remembered, it wouldn't be dead. Hurried up, I kept on dragging back. We had to go downstairs to a car the landlord had waiting for us, and now we were outside the flat, but the door was still open and I held back, looking over my shoulder as I was pulled away.

It was the last thing I saw, the fan on the living-room ceiling, my night-time friend. Waking up hot in the

night, getting out of bed and standing under it in the
dark, I had lifted up my arms to let it cool me. Listening
to it sometimes, speeding up and slowing down, the
whir of it pushing air through its big blades sent me
back to sleep.

The car's engine was running as I was pulled in; we
drove fast through the city, bumping on pavements and
swinging from side to side. Reaching the ship just in
time, we were the last on board. As the gangplank was
raised, people arrived on the quay: dozens of men
shouting, waving their fists and throwing things.

The lumps of iron and stone being thrown at the ship
were muffled as I went to sleep that night, like echoes
getting smaller and further apart. I floated away from
them, like the ship itself, away into a sea-deep sleep.

In the morning, the land had gone. There was miles
of sea – and another vicar to sort out for the return
journey.

'Hello' I said, walking straight up to where he was
sitting with his face to the sun. He made a place for me
by his side and I began to tell him the long version of my
story about God.

Years later, I saw how both my parents suffered from
our Egyptian stay. My father, who loved the RAF and
peacetime flying, did as his job demanded. Under orders
to stay in Nairobi, he came to rescue us when he could.
For my mother it had been too late. There were quarrels
on the journey back: over my father's job; where we

would live; what we would do.

On our return from Egypt, when I was six, first an incident in a London taxi, then a nightmare. In the taxi I was sitting between my mother and father. The argument was over me, this time, over who I should live with now that I was getting bigger. My father wanted me to go to him and be looked after by his mother in England, and my mother wanted me to be with her and her mother and father in Wales.

'She's coming with me.'

'No, she isn't, she's staying with me,' said the other, giving me a pull.

If I could have, I would have cut myself down the middle and given half for my mother and half for my father. For I loved them both. I loved the fun in my father, the trips to the beach, playing ball, running, swimming, splashing in the water and the presents he bought too. It was exciting when he came home.

Life with my mother was quiet. But I loved her too – and I was *her* child.

Stuck between them as they quarrelled, I knew I couldn't give them what they wanted. They needed me to be two children, one each, and I was only one.

The nightmare was this:

On a huge ship, there was the Captain, my mother and father and me. We were in the middle of a storm, wind and rain nearly pushing us over. The ship was like a galleon I'd seen in pictures, with big billowing sails. White horses in the sea were making it go up and down.

The Captain was fierce. He told me either my mother or my father had to walk the plank and I had to choose which one of them was going to die. They stood in front of me. Looking from one of my parents to the other, I couldn't do it. I would never be happy whichever way my finger pointed.

But however much I begged and cried the Captain wouldn't change his mind.

Someone in the family had to die.

Chapter Twelve

~§

NELLIE

On the thirty-five-mile journey back from visiting Renzo in Kent I feel trapped:

'Go away and think,' he has said. 'You have past injuries. Only you know what's in your life.'

And then another phrase:

'I can work on the muscles. Only you can work on the mind.'

But how? I have no idea what these past injuries are, or how to work on my mind to find them. If Renzo were anyone else, I would say he was wrong. One of us is. Where *are* these injuries? What will it matter if I find them or not? Frustration, despair.

While I accept the body and mind are bed-fellows not separate entities, I'm seeing Renzo for a physical condition – and the past, so heavy and present in me, can't be changed. I know the weight of it. It's where I spend my days; hours of sitting watching pictures;

weeks; months of them; me a living cinema. But where will it lead me? It seems pointless.

In my armchair seat I've seen a picture of the child on a shelf in a Sanderstead flat, carried down the years like a ship in a glass bottle. There's a lamp after this, an ornate, old-fashioned affair a genie might spring from. I know what it is, but had forgotten it. It's from the Middle East. Then there's an image from a photograph album, a black and white picture of my mother and father standing arm in arm in evening dress on board a large ocean liner, ready to go to the ball. Then one of my mother in the desert, one hand on her hip, the other shielding her eyes against the sun.

There's another child now. It's Victorian London, the mid-1890s, evening time. She is eight years old, sitting on a suburban train, clutching a rough bundle in her arms.

Anxious, she doesn't want anyone to know about the coins in the cloth pouch under her skirt: money to take home to her mother for rent, with whatever's left over for food. Pushing herself hard into a corner by the window, she fixes her eyes on the buildings outside, staring through the grime.

The bundle is heavy and she holds it close so as not to drop it. Back stiff, knees clenched, she is ready to hurl herself forward and run with it – home, home. But she must wait for her stop.

My father's mother, Nellie.

A sepia picture on the mantelshelf over my aunt's

hearth of a winsome, eighteen-year-old girl leads me to her story. I first remember her from the age of around four when, visiting her in the time we lived in the Sanderstead flat, I was left on her doorstep because she didn't like my mother and wouldn't let her in.

She was nice to me then. She showed me her wooden leg, although it wasn't all wood. Mostly made of tin, and almost to her hip, she got it after a bomb hit the gas cooker she was hiding behind in the war. Sometimes I watched her put it on after her afternoon rest.

My memories of the stump of her real leg are as clear as if Nellie were still here. It was skinny and milky-white until you got to the end, about six inches below the hip. There it was puckered and darker from being stitched. This end bit was like a scrunched-up face and it fascinated me, unlike the white bit, which was flaccid and vaguely disturbing.

Every day, Nellie fixed on the complicated wooden leg with its different-sized brown straps and buckles. The false leg had a hollow where the stump, washed and powdered, fitted in. It had a black tin bit for the calf, which was covered by a thick, grey-brown stocking, and a shiny black shoe at the end to match my grandmother's other one.

The shoes were like a man's: thick-rimmed, thick-soled lace-ups with a chunky, wedge heel. These, a walking stick, and the fact that the leg creaked, made sure you knew when Nellie was on the warpath. There was a thump when her stick hit the ground, then a series of squeaks and creaks, followed by a heavy footfall, then more thumps.

At night, she propped the leg up in the corner within reach of the bed so she could put it on in the morning. She also had a spare leg in a drawer of the tallboy. This spare one influenced me to lead a perilous childhood. For I believed God — who gave people their bodies — operated a spare parts factory in the sky, filled with replacement limbs made of tin just like Nellie's. Swinging from branches and jumping off high swings and walls, I called for other children to follow in my footsteps: 'You don't have to worry if you break something' I shouted. 'You can have spare ones.'

This is what I did when, as a six-year-old, after we came back from Egypt, Nellie lived with us. Her good leg painfully seeping shrapnel at the time, she needed care. We settled, the four of us, on an RAF camp in the Midlands, my father still flying. But not for much longer.

A daredevil at times, his plane did a deafening — and forbidden — loop-the-loop over our garden one sunny lunch-time and my mother could take it no more. Running in from the clothes line, she sat at the kitchen table and said: 'I can't stand it. This can't go on.'

My own life was impossible by this age. With quarrels in the house about my father leaving his job, of us going to Wales — or was it Surrey? — I struggled to find something to hold on to, something that wouldn't move or leave me

behind or be taken away from me. But I had to be good
at the same time – or sink.

A strict parent, which is what she thought you ought
to be, my mother had no patience for bad behaviour,
and she had thousands of other children to hold up to
me if ever I complained: all the children worse off than
myself who were starving in India, homeless in Africa,
hungry and orphaned and not lucky like me. How I
resented them.

I was unhappy too, at how the smiling, cheerful side
of my mother was kept for grown-ups outside our house.
With the woman next door she laughed a lot, but in our
place her smiles were shut away.

Over years of changes, in home circumstances,
schools and countries, I learned to fit in and adapt to
other people: to their habits and different needs of me.
I changed handwriting, table manners, accent and,
once, even my name – although that was a bid for
freedom in an African boarding school. I was twelve and
experimenting with the idea of being someone else.
Long before I set foot on African soil, I had become a
chameleon.

But with Nellie living with us, there was no hiding
place. She definitely didn't like me any more. And like
God, she had X-ray eyes that could see into the middle
of me, to the part where my den was, the place which
must be defended for me to survive. Nellie's eyes were
nasty places to fall into, like crocodile pools, and I
avoided her gaze as much as I could. If God had

hundreds of eyes, then Nellie's one pair was as bad as all His put together and, when she looked at me, I felt she had the power to make me vanish.

She used the same words as my father: 'Look at me when I talk to you, child', and that is what I didn't want to do. Looking at Nellie was risking death. So began my out-of-body experiences. They happened in the car. In the house, the noise of her wooden leg gave me time to escape. In the car, I couldn't get away from her.

I sat in the back seat. Nellie sat in the front while my father was driving. My mother stayed at home cooking and cleaning. I had to sit on the right-hand side so Nellie could see what I was getting up to. When I thought she wasn't looking, I turned my head to stare hard out of the window at the fields and trees and sky, and then the feeling of floating started.

When this happened, I put my hand carefully next to the door where she couldn't see. I rubbed my thumb and finger round and round and the space between them grew to the size of a football. Then bigger and bigger, much bigger than the car, and as big and round as the whole world outside. And I was gone away, floating up in the air.

I was brought down again by a voice from the front seat which sounded far away to begin with, and then nearer:

'Didn't you hear Nana talking to you?' my father would ask sharply.

The answer was 'No', but like many childhood truths,

it was more than my life was worth to speak it.

I was coming up to seven by this time, trying to form a picture of the world outside myself and how I fitted into it, and in my personal jigsaw, too many of the pieces were wrong or missing. My life was full of different people and strangers and objects which got lost and felt like bits of my life disappearing. Dolls and dolls' houses were left behind as we moved, or they were sold, or given away to other children, as were books, teddy bears, trinkets and clothes. All vanished: a fan in an Egyptian ceiling; other children in the different schools I went to. I was all at sea.

On one of our visits to Wales, when I was out playing with some other children in the street, I thought Harry and Bessie had vanished. All the semi-detached council houses with their red bricks were the same and when I searched for the one Harry and Bessie lived in, I couldn't find it. My sudden scream brought Harry flying out of a door only a short distance away from where I was standing.

My mother didn't help. She didn't take my side when Nellie told lies about me. Like my times in the Sanderstead flat, I was growing smaller again. I was afraid of things going away from me which I couldn't get back.

Struggling to survive on my own resources, I wanted to know with great intensity, and as if my life depended on it, which pieces of my life went where, and in what order. Did we go to Egypt before Wales, and how many times was Wales? My mother was worn down by it and sent me out to play.

I tried to compensate by reaching out and talking to people – and writing to them too – but I was unsure of the rules of engagement, so a kind grown-up who gave me a piece of chocolate on a train might well be asked for an address so I could write one of my letters.

By the age of eight, I had a growing correspondence with the outside world. I had attached myself to a number of children's magazines running correspondence clubs, and I sent off the poetry I wrote. Wherever I went, I carried a worn-down pencil or three behind my ear, in my pocket, cardigan sleeve or side of my shoe. Some days if you shook me you'd get a rain of stub-ends.

I waited for the postman the way other children waited for Father Christmas. If he didn't bring me a letter when I was expecting one, I sat in the field at the bottom of the garden looking for four-leafed clovers. When I found one I wished I had a baby sister or brother, or that Nellie would go back to her own house, or that I was somebody else's child, somebody who was nice to children. I thought if I huffed and puffed hard when I made my wish, I could make it happen.
By this time, my belief in my power to change things was enormous.

But I needed stamps for my letters, and my grandmother tried to stop my mother giving me them.

'I know I've already had one,' I said to my mother, trying not to cry. 'But I need another one to write to

Enid Blyton, and she'll be waiting for my letter, and she won't write back to me if I don't write to her first . . .'

Nellie said it was wrong for me to have letters to myself, and I was afraid she would steal them. Anxious around the house, I began to watch Nellie as she watched me. But then, relief. After three months my mother's hot poultices had worked. Nellie's leg was better. She was going away, back to where she lived in Surrey.

A change of home for us followed soon after. My mother's pleas and threats worked and my father left the Forces. We moved to Lincoln where he began working for a big engineering company.

But he didn't like his job.

In the decade or more which followed, looking for work that would make him happy, he went abroad. Sometimes he journeyed ahead of us, to find out if the new place was suitable for women and children.

Other times, we travelled with him.

Chapter Thirteen

ᵉ§

A WOMAN IN THE AIR

Sometimes seeing Renzo makes me despair. His insistence on the injuries in my past is about equal to my inability to find them. And there's something else he insists on: overworking is also a problem and I am trying too hard. I have to allow more time. But how? How can I stay connected to the real world and do nothing: shut away from reality, in a vacuum – or a pocket of time?

Returning to my armchair seat, the pictures, too, return. In the one of my parents arm in arm on an ocean liner ready to go to the ball, my father is in a dinner suit, and my mother, much shorter than him, is wearing a dress I remember from when I was nine years old. It is heavy, green taffeta, rich and, like her, rustling with light. Strapless and tight waisted, it falls away to layers of flounces swirling at calf level.

Oh, what a pretty dress. And, oh, how she danced in it: quick; deft; the heavy swish of the fabric trying to keep pace. She could tango, quickstep, foxtrot, rumba, waltz, cha-cha-cha or Highland Fling, my mother moving, the frock a step behind.

In the many big ships we travelled on together in my childhood there was a common greeting:

'Here's spring,' people would say as my mother entered a room.

'And here comes autumn.'

The latter was for my father, following behind her. Flying career over, trying to adjust to life on the ground, he was struggling: getting social events wrong; misreading them. Thinking it was jokes that were needed, women got drinks spilled on them and men too as my father 'accidentally' bumped into them. Tempers were tried – and shins too – for another 'joke' of my father's was to kick people lightly under the table and pretend it wasn't him. People felt uncomfortable, got embarrassed and, eventually, left.

My father's idea of fun wasn't the same as other people's.

Falling to my mother to take seriously the matter of my upbringing, doing her part on her own, as she saw it, she made sure I was clean, well-behaved – and grew up fast. The Future was a big thing with her and she propelled me determinedly towards it. From a four-year-old in Sanderstead with Time wrapped up in parcels, I was looking ahead, a girl leaning forward, seldom resting back.

My mother's will to urge me on in this way is as difficult for the shape of my life as the covered-up grief in my father. She fires in me a streak that is all go. I'm on blocks, waiting for the off, leaning on Time like there's no today – only tomorrow.

This is what I'm doing when, at the age of twenty-one, I become the youngest reporter the Manchester office of the *Daily Mail* had employed at that time. I am grabbing a new job, work, the future, as if my life depends on it. I'm running away from the past at full speed.

At night I was happy sitting in a bedsit in a suburb of Manchester, a city where I knew no one at all outside the office, in a room no more than thirteen or fourteen feet square. It had a chair, table, single bed and a wardrobe, and no one could get me. I wanted no more.

By day I was a news editor's gift: eager and petrified in equal measure. On a story I was like human blotting paper, absorbing what I heard or saw, then wringing myself dry to get it out of me again and on to the page. Then I did it all over again the next day and the next, and the month and the year after.

'I can do that' was my response to being asked to do something. But when a deputy editor suggested I take a few days off in lieu of the excessive hours I was putting in, I froze: 'What would I do with a day off?' Beyond the office in the big city where I lived, I knew nothing and no one outside an interview or a story. Work was what I knew, my success coming not from talent especially, but from exclusion – desperation to exclude the nightmare possibility of failure, of going back instead of moving on. If I lost my job I would have to return to my parents' home. Failure was the abyss.

So I worked. Other newspapers were combed, magazines and trade journals read, phones answered, contacts called and ideas put forward. After long hours in the office, the activity continued. Reporters stuck together in a drinking, nightclubbing, partying pack. There were birthday parties, leaving dos, celebrations for getting the front page lead, drinks all round for a new baby – and an intimate table for two now and then. But relationships weren't easy. Impossible to keep private, hit by round-the-clock shift patterns, they suffered a high casualty rate – and the office was never far away.

At night, someone would call in on the hour, tell the others what was going on. Whether needed or not, we would be back around midnight for the first editions, and then return from clubbing at two to cheer up the late duty reporters. If we were still out at three, we slumped down at a desk to begin the slightly drunken process of hatching a possible story for the next day's paper. Or else we followed up a police contact in the hope that he was off guard too.

It was a hard, frantic, exhilarating life and you paid a high price for it. I collapsed, just once: the beginning of a slow turning point, a shiny pivot inside my tight, frightened mind.

I'd been working twelve- to fourteen-hour days on a long series which was drawing to an end. The idea behind it was simple – and novel at the time: go under cover and write your story from the inside out. Instead of doing an exposé on beauty contests, I'd enter one incognito, and write about it first hand.

The first of these exploits came from a few paragraphs in an evening paper. The Territorial Army had a new training technique called paragliding – parachuting without jumping out of a plane. It was a way of training pilots how to fall properly from parachute jumps without the costly and time-consuming business of using a plane.

Instead of baling out, you sailed skywards from a standing position on the ground via a strong rope attached to a Land Rover at one end and a buckle on your waist at the other. A parachute lay draped behind you. When the Land Rover started moving, the rope tightened. You started walking to keep pace and, as air filled the chute, it took you up. When you were ready to come down, you released the buckle and descended into a fall.

The editor agreed this was an excellent wheeze for a young reporter – especially a female one – to try out, and to write about. The TA agreed, and a date was set for me to go up on a Sunday morning in May, with a large expectant hole in Monday morning's paper.

The exercise took place on an aerodrome runway. You were dressed in full flying gear: boots; helmet;

jumpsuit. The buckle for the rope hooked on to on your belt and the other end clipped to the back of a jeep some 1,000 or so feet away. The slatted parachute was draped from a harness on your shoulders ready to be filled up with air.

It must be said, no one on the airfield wanted me to go up: heavy winds were gusting up to gale force. But in simulated exercises on the ground, I learned how to fall from a standing position and was eager to test myself. It was the hole in the paper I was thinking of – and the chance of flying into page three or five. As it happened, I nearly filled a page near the back.

The near-fatal error was spotted within seconds of me leaving the ground: no one had thought to weight my parachute. Most of the TA men were big, around 15–16 stone. I was little more than half that weight. Without the extra ballast, I shot into the sky like a rocket, a before take-off smile for the cameras almost ripped off my face. Arriving breathlessly at around 1,000 feet, it took only seconds for an awful truth to hit me – I couldn't get down again. I was stuck in the sky.

High winds were keeping the rope between me and the ground taut as wire and you couldn't let go of the rope while it was taut. If you did, the sudden release of tension would act like a spring and send you somer-saulting – dive-bombing head first to your death.

I had been warned, of course, and ten seconds up, fervently wished I had taken heed. It could be a long time before the wind dropped – and I was fixed high in the air at the end of a jeep. From this height, vehicles look like Matchbox toys and people are little bigger than army ants. There's no hope of communication.

Other awful things were happening. I'd been told to avoid rocking backwards and forwards in case a sudden gust of wind flipped me over into that fatal somersault. But I was beginning to flap back and forth anyway, helpless as a bit of washing on a clothes line. My helmet was clattering non-stop with the force of the wind, and my head, ears, jaw and teeth were taking a battering.

I had not yet met the flying window cleaner, the man who had time to think how much it would hurt before he hit the ground. I kept on imagining how many bones I'd break in the crash earthwards – death even.

On the ground, people were waving their arms, trying to tell me something I couldn't fathom. I was relieved to recognise an ambulance coming along. Slowly, I began to understand what the ground crew was on about. The Land Rover was zig-zagging, trying to create some slack in the rope. None came. Then it began to twist round and round on its axis in a tight circle. Momentarily, the rope dipped slightly. What should I do?

The advice had been:

'There must be plenty of slack in the rope before you unclip the buckle, a good, deep curve.'

Dozens of people on the ground were waving things now – flags. But what were they saying? Were they telling me to take this small chance, to undo the buckle? Or were they warning me not to? I hesitated – and got it right. The warning was not to.

That moment passed. As did others, and I was tiring. My arms and legs were leaden, and the effort of keeping them wide apart in a gale was getting too much – like my clattering helmet.

The Land Rover continued zig-zagging, picking up speed, braking sharply, turning, until, near exhausted by this time, I saw a bit of slack. Was it enough? What were the waving flags telling me? My hand on the buckle, I unsnapped it and let go the rope.

The next ten minutes were extraordinary. Instead of landing somewhere decent on a nice piece of grass, I was heading for the woods – at a speed of close on 30 miles per hour. Land Rover and ambulance tailing me over rough ground at the wood's edge, I hit earth like a trouper: ankles; knees; hips; shoulders. No sickening snap of a bone, no pain, twist or wrench. But I was still moving.

Trees to my left, vehicles catching up to the right, the parachute, still lively and filled with air, was pulling me along at a good lick.

A few hundred yards further on, with the Land Rover alongside doing almost 20 mph, two men jumped out the back of it on to the frisky canvas. That was that. Everything stopped. A moment of astounding stillness, the world gone away. Then, things coming back at high speed and volume: voices, questions, hands on me.

With no broken bones in my body – and my head full of gales still – I refused to go for X-rays. Nothing hurt.

Why stop now? I also refused to lie down. Writing the article on the airfield, it was in the paper the following day – with a picture of me kitted out and soaring upwards. I was in the office.

Over the next few days and weeks my arms, legs and spine produced an amazing variety of red, orange, brown, purple, blue, green and yellow bruisings. The editor, meanwhile, was on to something. Could I do more of this kind of thing, he wondered.

'I can do that,' I replied.

The dozens of such articles which followed were met by radio interviews, TV appearances and job offers. But I was twenty-two, and hadn't a clue how to handle it. I stayed put with the *Mail*, not from loyalty especially, but from lack of imagination about what it would be like to leave.

The event which was to change all this happened in Conway, North Wales. Training with the Green Berets this time, the detail no one thought to check was if I could hold my own bodyweight with my arms and shoulders. I couldn't. As a child swinging from trees or exercising in the gym, I just hung there, then dropped. Yet the drill with the Green Berets involved being able to abseil down a 100-or-so-foot-high brick stack by holding your own weight.

You stood at the top of the stack with a strong rope wound intricately over your shoulder, round your waist, between your legs and into your hands. Taking a deep breath, you then jumped off the edge. Dangling, you were supported by this rope – and your ability to hold yourself in place on it. If you could do this, you let out a bit of rope at a time through your hands, and then bumped your way gently down the side, like you saw in adventure films.

The Green Berets were giving a public display that day, hundreds of people watching. The really scary bit was jumping off the top. The rest should have been easy . . .

Once over the side, the rope slid through my bare hands, burning them. I released my grip. But I was all wound up in a rope cradle, all of it sliding along my skin as I headed for the ground. Wearing only light cotton clothing which was singed through in a flash, this time I was mightily pleased to be taken to hospital.

Thanks to swift treatment no infection set in. Matron came to see me, though, as I lay on the ward, chastened and still trembling from the burns. She looked specially dressed up for the occasion in masses of starch, epaulettes and what appeared to be medals. She viewed me reprovingly.

'I've been looking at your picture in the papers,' she said in a prim Welsh accent. 'And with what you've been getting up to I was expecting to see you in hospital long before now.'

Chapter Fourteen

⌘

OLD INJURIES

When he's questioned me about previous injuries, I haven't told Renzo about the paragliding incident or this abseiling escapade. I've half-forgotten them. I tell him the next time we meet. I also tell him about another incident some years later when, drunk, a man pulled away a chair as I was about to sit on it and I landed on the floor, jarring my coccyx.

'So,' says Renzo, 'you had these two bad injuries—'

I interrupt:

'I didn't have to go to hospital. I didn't think they were serious.'

Renzo says he has treated a number of people who have landed on their coccyx. One is partially paralysed. *He* considers that serious.

He tells me the relationship between the cervical spine, in the neck, and the lumbar spine in the pelvis is finely balanced, one curve offsetting the next so that a blow to one is absorbed, like a shock wave, by the other.

'You had already hurt your neck with the paragliding,' Renzo says, 'and then you sit on the floor.' Then he asks: 'Were you trying to kill yourself –' he pauses – 'how do you say it in English? – on expenses?'

The same thought has occurred to me, going back over those reporting years from my armchair seat. There are various ways of being careless with a life and I'm shame-faced about all that bravado. I recall how driven and keyed up I was at the time, and the nights of lying anxiously awake wondering if I would fail the following day, wondering if that would be the day my world would fall apart.

Many times doing the series I got up at 5 a.m. to keep a 10 a.m. appointment 200 miles away because I was afraid of hotels and would rather get up at dawn than stay in one. Like a snail, I couldn't manage without the shell of familiar homely objects to sleep among: the protection of my own reading lamp; the pictures on the wall; the books; the pencils and pens in a pot. The woman who had her picture in the papers in the morning, who rocketed up into the sky and jumped off chimney stacks by day, was afraid to sleep away from home at night. But why was I afraid, not only of this, but of many other things too? Going to see a doctor about it once, nervousness is what I called it, but I didn't know how to explain. All I came up with was that however many times I did things, I was still nervous when I did them again. He didn't ask for details. Maybe I wouldn't have supplied them.

Going to work every day, I was taut, anxious. Every new story the same: a trial. In the office, tension rose in me as the news editor got up from his seat and walked towards the reporters. Then, a hand on my shoulder.

'Carol. This has come in. Take a look at it. We think the woman's in Sheffield. Her husband's gone to ground up in Cumbria somewhere. Get on the road and give us a ring in a couple of hours.'

Relief, then, to be doing something, but tension returning as I got under way, every car journey to every story a suspense. Would I get there in time? Would I miss something?

Perhaps sensing how fearful I was in the office, a senior reporter was kind: 'The day you're *not* nervous in this job is the day you're dead,' he said.

But I felt risen from the dead every morning. Each day I woke with the same anxiety that I wouldn't be able to cope and that the world I had built myself, of a life, a flat, a job, would disappear. So I was up within minutes of waking, reassembling myself as hard and fast as I could, starting from scratch, re-inventing myself from nothing.

The more I accomplished – standing up, stretching, getting dressed – the more of myself came back to me. Within ten minutes of getting out of bed, my first waking feelings were waning and an hour later they seemed like nonsense. The more things I put into the day as it rolled on – activities, work, chores – the further the morning's anxieties seemed to recede.

Going to bed at night, I believed I'd done it, put

myself back together for good. Lying in the dark before falling effortlessly into sleep, I believed I wouldn't crack apart this time, that I'd be held, whole, through the night. I'd done it at last. But no. Every morning I woke up, my achievements flown away from me in the dark. And it was in front of me again – this feeling of having lost myself.

What I was able to describe of this to the doctor was how nervous and unsure of myself I was. Was this normal I asked. He was avuncular, said he thought I was paying a price for being in a high-pressure job, said how much he enjoyed reading me in the paper. These kinds of anxieties were not uncommon in young people, he told me, and gave me some pills, telling me to come back if I didn't feel better.

When, after a few weeks, they didn't work I threw them away and relied more heavily on my job to keep me together and safe. Interviewing people on their doorsteps, sitting in their offices and homes, I put as much distance as I could between me and the falling-apart woman who woke each day.

Other people's lives were like a drug to me.

These images from the past continuing, Renzo tells me my body is still improving slowly. We are four months into treatment, and I'm almost a year into whatever has seized me. Within a short time I shall move to a new home. It's small, but has big windows letting in light in a street where there are plenty of trees.

I was beginning to fear it wouldn't happen, that I'd stay stuck for ever inside two rooms of a house which was once mine, and inside a body which was once familiar to me too.

Still no question of working, but I'm gradually exercising my way to regaining mobility in my neck. I have many small and irritating pains, but the Big Guns, the vice and the electric shock treatment are mostly silent.

As the pain has lessened, the relationship between Renzo and me has improved. It feels less dependent – less as though our sessions are all there is between me and despair. But it's still unbalanced, one where I lie down and a person who is standing up places his hands on me, week after week, while I hope for recovery. I rely on him and he doesn't rely on me. I'm corrected when I say this:

'An osteopath's job is to help the body to heal itself,' Renzo says. 'So we rely on the patient, first of all to allow this to happen, and then to tell us things, so we know what's happening in the body.' He smiles as he adds:

'And of course we have to know what the patient is hiding from us too.'

Our sessions mirror this. I explain what I think is happening to me physically and what I've noticed in the last week that might help him. He, in turn, examines my body to find out what I've not told him. He runs his fingers and sometimes the palm of his hand along my spine and shoulders.

'Ouch,' I'll say, as he touches one of my ribs or presses a shoulder blade.

After this, I lie down and he continues using his hands and fingers to knead or unknot various bits of my shoulders, back, sternum or neck. While it feels reassuring, it's still difficult to believe so little happens in these treatments. I yearn for more – a dramatic 'click,' perhaps, that will put me to rights. Instead he tells me to be patient, and to go away and think.

One day Renzo says:

'Your body will hold itself up by itself, you know. It will hold itself up without you doing anything.'

So that's what's happening! As soon as he speaks, I know it. I'm holding myself up as if I have to – a human hanger. I've had a life-long belief that it's my job to hold up my body. I thought that's what you did, made sure you kept it straight, like you were told. Now I see: it's what you do when you *don't* own one – when it's rented. God has been here all the time: you shall not breathe; you shall not be free; your body is not your own. That's the suit of armour – keeping myself rigid.

I'm silent. The shock's too much. Then it's despair. I might as well give up. A childhood silliness: my body on loan from God, and not really mine. An adult life in place long since and God, I thought, banished. But no. He's here, like hell in my ribcage.

Over the next few weeks Renzo continues his calm exposition of how I don't have to work to hold my body together, that it's designed to do this by itself. I can trust

it to hold itself up, he says. It was built for that, and I
don't have to worry about it. But I do – and I'm pleased
he goes away for a few weeks.

I was brought up to fight illness. I haven't known
another way. Now 'illness' is within all of me in the
shape of my father's wish to make me a perfect girl for
God. The cells of my body were invaded from the inside
long ago, before I remembered what it was like to be
free. So can I ever be?

During my armchair reading, there's a word in an old
medical book – 'affection'. It describes a heart complaint, a wounding in 'the body's most vigorous muscle',
where the heart is 'affected' by disease. I adopt the word
for a while and there's relief in turning away from Insult
and Iron Finger.

There's relief, too, in reading – and pictures. There
are many images in the armchair by now. A new one of
the inside of my body is another Victorian picture: an
underground workplace, like a subterranean factory,
except it's high as a cathedral, spacious, efficient and
clean. All the workers are children. There's water going
up and down in buckets, a well, a small water wheel, a
mill for grinding. There's industry, but no strain.

The children are capable and healthy. They're co-
operative: knowing their jobs, they get on with them and
don't get in each other's way.

They remind me.

Chapter Fifteen

⋘৯

A GIRLFUL OF CHILDREN

The industrious side of me where there was work and no strain belongs in Africa where I went, for the first time, at the age of nine. The place where we lived was Ncema Dam, an isolated spot more than forty miles from Bulawayo. There, my father was a power house super-intendent in charge of the electricity to a small, scattered community. Being driven to the dam in my father's jeep, my first feeling of Africa was sky, warmth, colour, space and freedom. There were orange, purple and red shades of bougainvillaea, jacaranda trees, canna, brightly coloured bushes and miles of air and sky.

There were only three houses at Ncema. Standing in their own grounds, they were hidden from each other by trees and shrubs. Up a track, half a mile from the road, ours was a thatched, whitewashed cottage surrounded by a vast, colourful garden. It stretched as far as you could see, off into shrub grassland, then up into the kopjes, the rocky outcrops, where the leopards lived.

It seemed like Eden but, when the first excitement of waking up in Paradise had passed, the problems began. Lonely and longing for company, I went to call on the neighbours. In the first house they wouldn't let me in because they were 'snobbish', my mother said afterwards, and our family wasn't good enough for them. That left one house to go – and there I met the devil. Mr van J had one leg – one of his eyes was missing too, with a black patch over it – and he hopped around the place on one leg faster than other people went on two. Crutch clamped under his arm, he bounded about using it like a gun to stab at you. His real gun leant in the crook of his arm. He shot first and asked questions afterwards. But he was all there was.

He hated black people and, I imagine, soppy Welsh girls who liked reading and writing poetry. Except, that is, soppy Welsh girls who could shoot straight. His house was full of guns and rifles, hundreds of them over all the walls in the living room, bedroom, study, hallway, and in all the cupboards too. Shooting was his favourite activity and, perhaps hoping to scare me, he gave me a .22 to hold. But I liked the rifle, so he took me outside and told me to aim at a target.

I hit it in the middle.

He thought it was a fluke:

'Are you sure you haven't used a gun before?' he demanded after half a dozen straight aims.

Shooting the target was easy. Few things in my life had been and I didn't know what he was making a fuss about.

I thought Mr van J was a bad man, but he taught me things my parents didn't know: how to clean and load the .22; how to shoot even better; how to carry a rifle; how to kill ticks with a lighted match without hurting the dog; how to catch a growling dog by the mouth; how to pin a snake. I liked knowing how to do things. He loaned me the gun and I oiled and cleaned it with a soft cloth so its light brown body glinted in the sun. I enjoyed sawing wood and having a screwdriver in my hand, mending fuses and putting things together.

I liked bedding fence posts into the ground; unrolling big stacks of wire to keep out the leopards; digging trenches in the chicken run to stop the mongoose; banging nails into planks for the big kennels he kept; training the new dogs; and falling over laughing when a boxer went doolally over a spitting cobra. It hypnotised him, and he whined in a high-pitched vacant-eyed way for days before coming back to his silly senses. But I didn't like being in the kitchen with my mother. There was nothing interesting to do and I wanted to be outside.

For school, I did a correspondence course, which was okay until I got bored. I sent work to a headmistress hundreds of miles away and did extra work to impress her – sent her writing and poems – and she never once replied. I hated her by post.

My mother, on the other hand, hated Africa. It wasn't clean enough, and I disobeyed her by bringing lizards and chameleons into the house. They lived in my bedroom, but sometimes they escaped. I liked having lizards around. They made life interesting. My mother did not.

So I became cheeky. One day over breakfast I saw one of my lizards on the curtain rail. I smiled, watching it running, then its body staying still, then its head turned sideways as somebody moved, ready to run again. My mother wanted to know what I was looking at, and I wouldn't say. Then I started laughing. I played jokes on her after that. Sometimes I looked over her shoulder when there wasn't a lizard there at all!

My parents were bad company – little conversation and, except for cards sometimes, no games or fun. Whenever I could I stayed in the garden, roaming its edges, searching shrub and grassland for animals to sit and look at.

Deer and antelope wandered freely, often coming up to the front lawn, and I adopted the orphaned klip-springer, dik-dik or impala left by Mr van J's shooting. He didn't care if there was a baby left behind when he shot the mother. So I stepped in.

With an old saucepan of mixed milk and water in my hand, I went off to the garden's edge and watched for movement in the bush where the orphan had skittered off in fright, put the saucepan down and sat and waited. Often I was rewarded, and would slowly coax a young trembling impala away from the grassland up near the house where I could feed it without worrying about snakes. The snakes were all over: curled round the canna outside our window, and sliding across the small paths through the grass. But on the flat lawn, you could see them.

After adopting my young charge, I looked out every day for the flick of a tail, twitch of an ear, or the gleam of a glistening snout in the dry grass. Would it be behind a tree today, down by the chicken coop, up near the rocks? Sometimes I looked for miles and returned home to find it standing on the lawn waiting for me.

But I wasn't an African child yet, and I took the result of a leopard's night-time visit personally: one evening an impala; next morning a pile of bones. I was upset and angry.

The explanation which followed was garbled. My mother played no part in it, for she had wiped her hands of Africa. She was fighting colonies of ants in the food cupboards, a snake in the bathroom one night, another one which nearly killed our gardener, Walter, as he stood with his back to it chatting to her one day and she glimpsed it behind him, and my lizards and chameleons. When the impala bones were discovered, as far as my mother was concerned, that was Africa for you.

So my father had a go. I got an account which began with the impala having gone to an animal heaven in the sky where God was looking after it. I shifted awkwardly from foot to foot. This was followed by something to do with a food chain, and Mother Nature being unpredict-able about who ate what.

'Just like a woman,' my father said.

As the man in charge of the electricity, one night, for a joke, my father threw the switches and plunged us into darkness. I screamed. African bush nights are black, especially with a big thatched roof over your head, and I screamed again as he came from outside, making scratching sounds and ghost noises, and pushing the doors to make them squeak on their hinges. My mother was angry and shouted to him to stop.

Laughing about it the next day, he said she had no sense of humour. Then he did it again — and again. Around eight o'clock at night — my bedtime — he would throw the switch and come through the house and creep up on me. When I was almost breathless with fright, he stopped.

My father's joking was beginning to distress me.

The garden by day looked different too. Months had gone by and I was getting lonelier. There were no other children. I didn't want to feed any more dik-dik to make them into leopards' dinner, and I was bored. I hated the headmistress I never saw and all the dogs, Mr van J's and ours, weren't enough company.

I started making up plays and concerts. After my schoolwork, which was easy, I went to the trunk of spare clothes, got dressed up and pretended to be acting. Sometimes I was a pirate, and then I stopped doing that in case Mr van J got angry with me for copying him.

Sometimes I was a bride, which was easier but boring. After the fun of getting dressed in a satin cloth tied up with ribbons and velvet belts and draping a shawl over my head, there was nothing else to do. Other days, I walked round with a gun.

Wandering round the garden in wedding gear one minute and a gun slung over my shoulder the next I thought about God, and what my father said about God and Mother Nature, and I believed they were married and Adam and Eve were their two children. God was more important of course, like my father was more important than my mother, but Mother Nature made things happen too in the food chain, like my mother in the kitchen.

Thinking these kinds of thoughts, skipping for a bit, then sighing to myself, I made up a playmate, a boy Adam for my fed-up Eve. I showed this friend of mine flowers and oddities in the garden, shared with him information about Africa as if I had lived here for years, and invented games where I hid things in the bushes and trees and left written clues along the way for my playmate to discover. If he had difficulty finding a scrunched-up clue hidden in a tree stump or behind a piece of fencing, I would be patient for a while, and then, I'd say:

'Do you give in?'

He did of course.

'Here it is,' I exclaimed, pulling the piece of paper out of its hiding place.

But I wasn't the only person going mad. After six months, loneliness was tormenting my mother too and she called a halt. She told my father he had to find another job – in a place with people in it. Or else.

We left a few months after but before going, an event, a memory which I treasured. As with Egypt, it made me hold on to a place where I had been unhappy.

Exploring at the edge of the hill one day, I saw Walter, our gardener, in a clearing in his usual position, sitting on his haunches, arms on knees, twiddling a thin stick. He was waiting for his cousin, though I didn't know this at first. What I saw was Walter slowly stand up when he heard a lorry stop on the road way below and watch a man jump down from the back of it to begin the long walk up towards us. You could tell by his movements and the serious way he held his head and back straight that the man knew he was being watched and waited for – and Walter didn't wave or move.

When his cousin reached the clearing, Walter still stayed where he was and they stood for a few minutes, yards away from each other, looking, speaking a little, their eyes smiling, first their heads beginning to wake up, then their shoulders, arms, hands, legs and, eventually, feet. They still waited, eyes holding, walking almost on the spot, then round a bit, circling, till at last they were close enough to hug each other.

I knew I was seeing something important. Walter had waited months for his cousin to arrive, yet he stayed still, nothing thrown away, a slow remembering. It stayed with me: my first meeting with recognition.

Soon after, I was told I would have to leave Africa altogether because there wasn't a proper school at Mwadui in East Africa where we moved for my father's new job on a diamond mine. I would go back to Wales to live with Nana and Daddy Williams.

Dismay. I'd never stayed with Nana and Daddy Williams by myself. I didn't like the thought of it. I liked it in East Africa and wanted to stay. I had freedom out in the sun and in the mornings I went to a place where there were other children in a school of sorts where two teachers did games and lessons. Then I went home on a bus and I had a dog called Pal, an Alsatian. He met me every day at the school stop. When the bus came round the bend I watched his ears, like a rabbit's, bouncing through the long grass, telling me he was coming.

I had him from a puppy, and trained him so he sat still at the bus stop and I was proud of him when the other children saw what a good dog he was. Then, when the bus had gone, I let him jump all round me and bark how pleased he was to see me. After lunch, and the boring time when I was supposed to have a rest, he and I went out to look for creatures in the bush. We watched snakes and scorpions, lizards and geckoes, spiders and ants, vultures and African starlings, and he didn't move if I told him not to.

He knew how I was feeling. If I was angry, he walked

seriously by my side looking worried. If I was sad, he put a paw on my lap, and licked my hand. If I wanted to play, he jumped round me, then listened for what I told him to do. 'What's next?' his expression said.

I was nearly ten and I was many children: a dog-owner who knew how to train an animal; a mother to various orphaned antelope; an amateur electrician; a fence-maker; a good shot with a rifle; a sharp pair of eyes in the bush; a poet; a singer and dancer; a reciter of verse. A Welsh, English, African child.

On the outside I was a girl who didn't make a fuss and did as she was told. On the inside, Africa had grown in me, and I was big, and I didn't want to leave my dog. I'd parted with too many things before, in Egypt, and in places we moved on from, and he meant more to me than the books and toys I'd so often had to leave behind. If only he could come to Wales with me, it would be all right. Then I'd have a friend. But I was told I knew about quarantine, which I did, and Nana and Daddy Williams didn't want a big dog in the house and that was that.

The night before going to Nairobi to travel in a plane to Wales, the girl who does as she is told, and hides her hurt, puts on a concert for her mother and father. If they can't make it all right for her, then she must make it all right for them.

She goes to the kitchen cupboard and fetches a big broom. Her parents roar with laughter as she races round the room sweeping with it and making up songs and rhymes:

> 'Oh my, oh my,
> a piece of pie.
> Under the settee,
> Oh, woe is me.
> Naughty, Naughty
> Bad, bad, bad dirt.
> I'll smack and sweep you till you hurt . . .'

The broom sweeps, the child chants and the parents laugh.

Arriving by myself at Heathrow Airport late one winter's night, a few weeks after my tenth birthday, there was no one there to meet me. The airport was empty except for two women, an air and a ground stewardess, standing behind a desk. I wanted them to come and sit by me, but they didn't. Being impenetrable grown-ups, they let me sit by myself. Although, to be fair to them, I was by this time an awesomely composed child – at least on the outside.

I wondered how far Wales was. Had I ever known where Wales was, or was it one of those things I had forgotten in my time in Africa? But Africa was a long way away . . .

While I was asleep, Nellie arrived to collect me. It was

the middle of the night and she was in a bad mood. The next day, she put me on a train to Swansea, with a label pinned on me saying who I was and where I was going. I didn't like it, but I didn't take it off.

Nellie wasn't to be disobeyed, even at long distance.

Chapter Sixteen

ॐ

MY TIME AS A BOY

High summer has passed and just over a year into incapacity, I respond well to the flat of Renzo's hand urging my sternum to let go and allow me to breathe. He tells me I have 'exaggerated' curves in my spine, a pronounced S-shape in the cervical and lumbar regions. These have thrown my chestbone out, stopped me standing and breathing well.

He talks about his children, and we laugh as he describes how his son believed *he* was the father of his small sister when she was born and bossed his mother around.

I think about boyhood and, in the armchair, in my afternoons of 'diving', I retrieve the part of my childhood when I, too, was a boy.

Arriving in Wales a few weeks after my tenth birthday, after Nellie met me at Heathrow and put me on the train, I would not see my mother again for two years. I had been abandoned. My dog, Pal, was gone from my life too, and our afternoons together finding creatures in the bush. I moved from light, from the high days of an East African summer, where the sky had no limit above and around me, to a dark enclosed Welsh winter.

I wanted, more than anything, to tell the story of my African life, to shine it and keep it bright and clear in the box where I kept my memories. I wanted someone with Walter's eyes to greet me.

'Did you have a dog, what was his name, and what did you do together?' were questions I fantasised in my head – which is where they remained.

It would happen in all my moves. As I went from one place to another, my life had no adult witness, no one to confirm where I had been, what I had done, and help me keep its details safe. Memory was like a snake s-bending along the lawn then disappearing: heads; tails; vivid then gone. The box where I kept it was full of beginnings, endings; a child in a hallway knocking on closed doors. Becoming a boy for a year was what I came up with to cope with the door marked puberty.

Adolescence was something I hadn't been prepared for, had no knowledge of, and had not imagined. I knew there were grown-ups and children in the world. I thought you got from one to the other by getting bigger. I hadn't wondered how.

But before puberty, as I tried to have a life in Wales without my mother's shelter, there were other children to deal with. They asked me questions about myself: Who was I? Where had I come from? What was I doing here? Who did I live with? Why was I in Africa? Who did I live with there? Why did my parents send me away?

Adults' questions were difficult in a different way. They had lions on their mind – and black people: How many lions had I seen? How big were they? Did they eat people? Did black people wear any clothes? Was I frightened of them? Did *they* eat people? etc. These were the wrong questions and I didn't know how to answer them.

But in a small Welsh village a tall, brown girl from Africa was like a Martian, and my life was also exotic. I used the attention to tell the crowds who gathered to hear me speak from the school wall that I was going to be a film star because they travelled around and had their picture taken. I'd already had my picture in the paper in Africa – for being a white child stepping off a ship with a big doll in my arms. I was going to make a career of it, I told the playground throng – having my picture taken and moving on.

The true stories of my African life – the girl with the dog, and the child who stayed still, watching for movement in the bush – couldn't be told. In Wales, my life was an explanation, not a story, and, slowly, I lost the African pictures in it.

Another big change between Africa and Wales was the state of my grandparents' house. Cleanliness was a religion with my mother, as God was with my father. But in Harry and Bessie's place, neither God, nor a clean surface, was given the time of day. Bessie hated cleaning and tidying, dusting and polishing, and the housework was left undone.

The house being dirty made me squeamish. So did the 'black pads'. You didn't see them in the day, but if you switched off the lights after dark, out they would come, up from the mine shafts beneath us, hundreds of black beetles. If you crept down from your bed in the middle of the night to go to the outside toilet, you would see the floor covered with them scuttling for safety when you switched on the light.

Six of us lived there: Bessie and Harry slept in one bedroom; my two younger uncles, who had both just started working down the mines, slept in another; then us two children – my cousin Derek and me – slept at the back. My uncles teased me because I had an English twang and funny ideas about wanting clean towels.

I went to the local primary school, and it was there, one day, in those difficult early weeks in my first Welsh winter that it all got too much for me. I was sitting at the back of the classroom in a desk by myself, enjoying the warmth from the radiator and being in a proper school again, when huge frightening snakes came to get me.

One minute I was sitting still, the next I was being devoured from the inside by these creatures who were in my stomach. I wriggled a bit but it was no use, I couldn't get away from them. They were getting bigger

– giant cobras. They were going to swallow me up – and I'd be all gone.

Good girl though I was, I couldn't keep still with this lot in me. Leaping to my feet, I screamed and ran from the classroom out into the school grounds, fleeing for my life. I had done a few laps of the playground, running out of my skin with fear, before the snakes were quiet again and I could begin to be calm enough to think. I knew I would have some explaining to do when I was caught. But how? What would I say? I couldn't tell the truth. No one would believe I was being chased by giant cobras. Until I could come up with something, I kept on running. But what could I say instead?

I was on my fourth circuit of the playground by now, and the headmaster had been called. If anyone could catch me, he would. He was a rugby player: big, strong – and fast. It wasn't until the Head's heavy footsteps and strong breathing were hard on my snake-flying heels that I knew what I had to do.

Just at the moment he pounced, I let him catch me, then fainted in his arms. I was wide awake, however, behind my closed eyelids, but having shut them, I didn't know when to open them again. So, I kept them shut while the Head carried me to his car, drove me to 77, took me through the front door, up the stairs to the front bedroom, and into bed.

Then I must have fallen asleep, for when I woke, cautiously peeping out through lowered eyelashes to see what damage I had brought upon myself this time, I was surrounded by my own wake. Old women I'd never seen before were sitting round the bed, silent, except for the occasional shuffling noises they made. Some of them were rocking, some of them cried softly into their handkerchiefs. They had come to watch me dying.

Malaria is what the doctor pronounced on this occasion, shaking his head solemnly over my inert – and sleeping – body.

Round the village the news had run on the teacup trail, in and out of people's sculleries, up and down cinder paths, jumping over garden fences:

'Harry and Bessie's granddaughter has got a terrible disease with a funny-sounding name from Africa. Come quick!'

A few days after this episode, my grandmother found an unexpectedly practical streak in her fey nature: 'Malaria, indeed! Missing her mother is what she is,' she declared as I lay, speaking to no one, curled up like a large cat in the big chair by the fire. I cried then – for days. Eventually, this got up an uncle's nose: that, and me hogging the best chair in the place;

'Cry-baby, cry-baby,' he mocked, pulling a face at me.

When I got up and went back to school I didn't think about my mother any more. She was far away, and I would have to have my life by myself.

I was cheered by spring and fine weather arriving. One day, Derek was standing on the back step practising aiming with his catapult at tin cans on top of the post in the middle of the clothes line. I wanted to have a go too, but he wouldn't let me because I was a girl. But when his friends came, their aim was hopeless, and I made them give me a try.

Down came the can.

Up the line post went the boys.

Ping! Down came the can again.

No one in Wales knew about me learning to shoot in Africa. They'd have thought I was telling lies. But word soon got round there was 'a dab hand on tap' and by the following day, the Top-of-the-Suburbs boys' Gang, which Derek belonged to, had me in for auditioning. Via Derek and his mates, my reputation had preceded me, and when they saw how tall I was too, they forgot I was a girl.

'Crikey,' one of them said, blowing his cool. 'She's the best we've got, mun.'

Once having been formally adopted through an initiation ceremony of Chinese wrist twists, I became their chief stone-slinger in catapult contests with neighbouring tribes, of which the chief was the Bottom-of-the-Suburbs Gang. This lot had sand kicked in their faces — by a foreign girl. What a triumph for our lot! Although 'girl' was soon a banned word. The Top-of-the-Suburbs Gang fiercely defended my honour — my boyhood. Anyone who called me a girl after that got what for.

My pigtails were a nuisance, but I wore a flat, peaked cap over them, dirty jeans and jumper, and you never would have known there was a girl underneath. I begged

Bessie to chop off my plaits, but she wouldn't do it with my mother not around, although my aunt did – the one who was jealous of my mother – with some blunt kitchen scissors.

The suburbs in Trimsaran were surrounded by trees at that time. There was a big field at the bottom of the long gardens, and then, down a steep bank beneath that, thick woodland, and beyond that more fields and more woodland, and the occasional scattered farmhouse leading up into the hillside. It was a great place to run away from being a motherless girl, from the early beginnings of puberty, from the snakes and from God.

Our main stamping ground was the woods beneath the field at the bottom of the houses. We attacked them like locusts. A tree could be minding its business one minute, and the next, it was alive with flying, dangling, chattering bodies swinging off ropes, shouting, soaring through the air from branch to branch. When not up in trees, we swarmed the ferns like bees looking for something to attack. We swished sticks, stamped on brambles, jumped ditches and smacked the world. A fence, a stump, a bramble, a branch, a stone, a tree, a hill in our way, we smacked it.

Harry was a bonus. When he called us back at night from the woods, he didn't shout for us, he whistled by putting two fingers in his mouth and blowing. The whole gang looked up when this whistle came in the dark, like an owl calling. Then they looked at Derek and me and you could hear them thinking:

'Oh, to belong to a man who can whistle like that.'

And belong to Harry we did. Off we set, racing as fast as we could, falling in and out of ditches, flying up the bank, stumbling over tree roots in the dark, falling over ourselves to be first boy in. Breathless and almost giddy, we still put on an extra spurt at the garden gate and pushed each other aside to sprint up the long cinder path to be the first to reach him. You would have to see the proud look in our grandfather's smiling eyes to know why we, and any other child who knew him, flew to Harry like moths to a lantern.

I, with my flickering story and hidden lights, loved my Welsh grandfather.

Sometimes, in winter, when I was afraid to go to the outside toilet because of the dark, Harry would stand on the back doorstep waiting for me, whistling a tune to let me know he was there. Other times, he brought stout back from the pub for Derek and me as a special treat. The three of us stayed up late and Harry told us stories in the kitchen — big ones and small ones, fat and thin ones, old and new, all shining and polished.

Derek, being nine months younger than me, would begin to fall asleep sitting up, his eyelids drooping. Then up he'd jerk again, eyes open wide, and he'd stare at us, but without seeing. Down his eyelids would come again, then up and down a few more times before they stayed closed.

Harry wrinkled his nose at me and we smiled at each other to see how comical it was, Derek falling asleep, sitting up, in his chair.

Chapter Seventeen

✥

RELUCTANT LADY-DOM

I wonder about Renzo's son. He is ten, I find out, dark like his father, protective towards his sister and, I imagine, serious.

As Renzo talks about the strain in my body from a long way back, I tell him one day about my time as a boy: using a catapult, climbing trees, racing around. He looks puzzled. Then I realise why: I've used the word 'tomboy' and he doesn't know what it means.

I spent a spring, a summer and part of a winter hiding in boys' clothes, throwing stones, climbing trees, running, jumping and smacking the world. Then the catastrophe happened and I could hold back the future no longer. It was soon after the Christmas I turned eleven, and I fell from the high branch of a tree. Nothing unusual about that. The trick was to land on a lower and thicker branch. But I landed on my chest and there was no more ignoring the breasts that had been developing against my fervent wishes. The fall hurt fiercely, like a burn. I stayed still too long and the others knew. They were quiet in the rest of the tree, and when I dropped to the ground I knew I wouldn't be playing with them any more. It was over.

Calamity followed calamity. Within weeks of leaving the gang, Harry stopped me having a bath with Derek, and told me I couldn't have our special Saturday night treat any more. This was when Derek, he and I slept in the big feather bed together while Bessie went to Derek's and my room to snore through the night. Then he stopped me sleeping with Derek, and my uncles wouldn't talk to me because I was given their big room at the front – which I didn't want – and they had to have bunk beds in Derek's room. I created a hell of a stink, but Harry wouldn't give in. He said I had to sleep on my own because I was soon going to be a lady.

'But why do I have to sleep by myself because I'm going to be a lady?' I demanded.

'Because ladies don't sleep with their grandfathers and cousins,' was Harry's reply.

'But I don't want to be a lady,' I wailed. 'I want to sleep with you.'

I was furious. I wanted to go back to the woods, to climbing trees and making dens and belonging. Lady-dom was as appealing as falling in a bed of nettles. And it didn't get any better. Mourning my straight, uncomplicated boy's body, I was appalled at the ungainly, bow-shaped one which grew on top.

Someone, a cousin I think, said not to let a boy touch you 'there' once you started your periods, but why would a boy want to? Surely he'd never be that stupid. I had also heard tell that a boy knew when you were 'on'. Well, it was hardly surprising, given all the distress it caused. This is the kind of torment my father must have meant when he warned me before I left Africa never to let a boy touch me in a rude place or I'd burn in hell for ever.

God made a big comeback at this time via the Plymouth Brethren. For something to do, I went to their Sunday school. They talked about God like my father did. Only they had a way of avoiding the terrible business of a life of sin with an eternity of being damned at the end of it. You could be saved. So I was. They said I had to save other people too because everyone who wasn't saved would go to hell and burn.

Derek didn't want to know; my grandparents, not realising the way God loomed in my life, thought I was going through a silly phase; my uncles scoffed. But I was hooked.

Remaining in East Africa, on the diamond mine in Mwadui, my parents were in the middle of a two-and-a-half-year contract, or 'tour', at this time. They did three of these in all, with around three months' 'long leave' at the end of each one. They wrote fortnightly and one morning a letter arrived from my mother with the really amazing news that I had a baby brother. It was a surprise to everyone. No one knew she was having a baby. She'd been very ill, and the baby had too, but they were getting better now. He was six weeks old and before he was very much bigger, she was going to bring him to Wales for us all to see him.

Symmetry at last. I had never wanted to be my parents' only child. I was so excited I walked four miles to my aunt's house to tell her the news. But then I started to worry, and when I told the elders at Sunday school what I was worried about, they agreed with me. If he wasn't saved, my baby brother might die and go to hell before I even met him – and my mother too.

A child who didn't know her limits, my solution was logical – and off the wall. I would become a missionary and go back to Africa as fast as I could and rescue them both. Only one thing stood in the way – appendicitis.

I'd heard grown-ups in the kitchen saying someone had died of it. I didn't want this to happen to me on my way to Africa, so I prayed hard to have my appendix out. Even more bizarrely, the Brethren joined me in this prayer, and within months of it first being uttered, I was lying in an ambulance, its bell clanging as I was raced to hospital with suspected peritonitis. It was just before my twelfth birthday and there was snow on the ground. Perhaps we had all prayed too hard.

But it achieved an unexpected result. Thinking I might really die this time, my grandparents sent for my mother and she arrived within days – with my brother in her arms. He was nine months old by this time. It was love at first sight, and it was mutual. He believed in me and I believed in him.

A few weeks after my mother's return, when I was out of hospital, and lying on the settee in 77, recovering, there was a knock on the front door. It was one of the Brethren leaders. My mother was in the house next door having a cup of tea and, without thinking, my grandmother let him in.

My mother had banned me from having anything more to do with the Brethren. She told me what they said wasn't true, that it was all nonsense, and I didn't have to believe them. But within minutes of his kneeling by my sickbed, I was trapped again as the elder prayed to the Lord to rescue me, his lamb gone astray, from the clutches of the devil.

At that moment, in walked the devil herself – my mother. She had found the use of her English tongue in her years away and could stand up to people now.

'Who let you in?' was her first salvo to the large man struggling to his feet.

My grandmother, who had been bringing up the rear, scuttled back to the kitchen again, fast as a black pad.

'And what do you think you're doing kneeling by my daughter's bed?' my mother continued. 'Haven't you and your lot made her miserable enough already with your nonsense about hell and damnation? You should be ashamed of yourself, a grown man . . .'

The elder, who was more than a foot taller than my mother, tried to quash her with his superior gender and imposing stance, but she wasn't intimidated.

'If a group of men can't find better things to do with their time than prey on children in the street while their parents' backs are turned . . .'

'Now, come, come, Mrs Lee, in the name of the Lord, this is blasphemy . . .'

'I'll show you blasphemy,' roared my mother. 'You pick on a child when her parents are abroad, and nearly kill her with some kind of religious mumbo-jumbo about having her appendix out. What kind of behaviour is that? You're lucky I don't call the police. Now, get out of this house, and don't let me ever catch you talking to my daughter again.'

My brother was walking and a lovely springtime followed. I was beguiled by his smiling face, happy nature and the way he trailed round after me. He was my ally and I was proud when Harry called him my shadow.

My mother saw to it that the kitchen-table hair-chop my aunt had given me was tidied. I had a shaped cut which was called 'Italian Boy' and, with my thinness from being ill, probably that is what I looked like. She also helped me choose some new clothes. They included my first grown-up suit: a lightweight weave in grey and white with a simple jacket and a straight skirt. It made me look eighteen.

Most places I went my baby brother came too, either following behind or carried in my arms and when I wore the suit, which I did often, I was ever so proud when people thought he was mine.

But we were on the move again. The next East African contract was about to begin. That spring, all of us departed for Mwadui on another big ship, the Braemar Castle. I was glad to be leaving the Plymouth Brethren, cramped house, long dark winters and rain. A sea journey with dances, games, fancy dress, laughter and people to meet was just what I needed. I looked forward, as well, to the journey's end: a return to sunshine, open spaces, and, with my brother's arrival, a fantasy of family life.

But the adolescent girl who left Wales had accumulated a number of problems. If you counted the trips to and from her grandparents', she had been moved dozens of times at this point and the snaking thread of her life, its history and continuity, was jumbled up in knots and unsorted loops inside her. Yet she thought she was impervious to trouble and that with her brother by her side she could take on the world.

She didn't know it would take more than her brother's smile or her mother's dismissal of the Plymouth Brethren to protect her from a God who was already growing in her mind and body as swiftly as she, herself, was pushing forwards into the future. Neither did she know that the tension in her from a long way back was gathering like storm clouds and she was not out of the woods at all.

Chapter Eighteen

❧

THE SCHOOL WITH NO MIRRORS

As autumn settles in, Renzo talks his way round my body. Defiance of authority is in my chest, high up in the plate of bones he presses down on. He tells me about my body's defensiveness and about the slight deformity in my shoulders caused by muscles in distress pushing bones out of balance, not allowing them to settle.

The treatments have fallen into a pattern by now. The pains are familiar – except the ones I don't feel until his fingers touch them. I've stopped asking why he makes these probes along my vertebrae and shoulders because the answer is always the same: he is measuring tension.

I don't understand this because I can't feel it. When Renzo talks about deep tension in my thorax around T3 or T4, it doesn't make sense to me. I believe I'm defending a fortress and can spot the *obvious* tension by this time, relaxing my shoulders when I find them bunched up round my ears. But I can't feel the *deep* tension and undo my prison bars from the inside.

My first glimpse of the prison *inside* me was womanhood, a lonely and isolating state. Unlike the busy, exciting outdoor life of being a boy, being female seemed dull and restricting – a bleak prospect. At twelve, my touchstones were not promising: a Welsh grandmother who, wanting to be a concert pianist, resented the drudgery of cooking and housework; an absentee mother; and Nellie bearing me bad tidings with her wooden leg, X-ray eyes and gothic form.

But the big mail ships of the Union Castle line were magic places. As we left Wales in the spring of my thirteenth year, the cliffs of Dover were barely a blob on the horizon before I was taken aside. On deck, a girl called Bernadette, small, dark and dressed like a boy, told me the facts of life: ladies; gentlemen; bits; pieces; thingummies; what-nots; mens' bits going in wrong places; womens' bits being shocked; horror; farce; drama; calamity; hospitals; flower shops; jewellers; babies. I didn't believe a word of it, of course, but it was the start of my first proper friendship with another girl. We wrote and sent pictures of ourselves to each other for a long time afterwards.

Onboard ship, we talked about the grown-ups from our rail-side position, comparing and criticising: so-and-so's dress was too long; a man was too fat for his suit;

her hair was dyed; *she* wore pongy perfume which made us feel sick; *he* was after that woman; look, her eyebrows were painted. Sometimes we said nice things too.

I wore my new clothes on the ship: smart shorts; short-sleeved dresses and a red rock 'n' roll skirt. Middle-aged married couples who sat at table with us made a fuss of me and paid me compliments – which I'd never had before – and some officers taught me to rock 'n' roll.

At one stage, the ship's chaplain approached me to attend church and, not wishing to be rude, I gave him my latest, and most lengthy, version of the God story. I'd gone to church for a long time, I explained, but then God had made me miserable when my parents were in Africa, and I'd had to have my appendix out and . . . The chaplain beat a hasty retreat: the first sea voyage where I didn't take up with a vicar.

My father, it turned out, had put him up to it – to try and get me back to God. It's when the rows began between us: my father wanting me to be religious and it feeling like death to me. I'd just got away from the Plymouth Brethren and anything to do with God threw me into a panic. It was easy to avoid my father on a big ship – and I did.

Some weeks into the trip I got myself kissed. We were on deck at the time, briefly alone in between dances. I thought he was handsome in his uniform – tall and slim with dark hair and serious blue eyes; and just like the books said would happen, I went dizzy, weak at the knees, saw stars, sighed, almost fainted in his arms – and then did two full laps of the deck for fear of it happening again. It wasn't allowed.

But Africa was. As we reached its southern coast, I sensed the smell, the colours again, sharp, clear sounds carried through the air, sun shining on the water, busy quaysides, and imagined African ground beneath our feet. Holding my brother up over the rail as we came into port, we shared the excitement of being home again.

My brother was born in East Africa, where we were sailing towards, at Mwadui, a diamond mine ninety miles south of Mwanza on the southern tip of Lake Victoria.

Our home, Williamson's Diamonds, was built from sparse bushland by a Canadian geologist, John Williamson. As a young McGill graduate, he dreamed of finding gemstones in this part of the Shinyanga plains and, against advice, ill health and the spoiling tactics of diamond moguls De Beers, he did so.

Staking his claim to the ground, trees were planted, houses and roads built, an airfield and an infrastructure to support a thriving mining community – a workforce, huge by bush standards, of a hundred or more European families and many more Africans. At one time, one of the richest men in the world, he gave away diamonds as gifts – a famous blue for Princess Margaret, but he left before the Royal plane flew in.
Shyness.

It was a long train journey inland to this, our home,

and within a few days of arriving, I was on my way again, on another train with a hundred or so other teenagers, to a make-shift boarding school called Kongwa. I don't recall what I felt about leaving so soon, but I remember the excitement of driving out in the bush at night to catch the train. You boarded at midnight, miles away from where we lived, on a bend in the track where, if you signalled with a lantern, the train slowed down enough to let you on.

Standing by the Land Rover, waiting in the dark, with animal sounds close by, the deepness of the night – miles of it – held me. I felt safe. At the boarding school I was heading for, I got into trouble for this, for wandering in the dark, climbing trees and listening to the night.

It was a two-day trip to Kongwa, and since it wasn't the beginning of term yet we did what we liked. We stayed awake late just because we wanted to and to hang out of windows finding animal shapes in the dark. Propping each other up in the small hours, we told each other true stories about ourselves which we wouldn't have said in daylight. When someone dropped off, we rearranged a book, arm, leg or blanket.

At the end of this journey was the hot, dusty interior of unending bush. Kongwa School consisted of leftover Nissen huts, home to a few hundred children and numerous insects, snakes, scorpions and hyenas. Mostly, things like snakes stayed outside – sometimes in the loos – but you could never be sure.

The showers were outside too, next to the loos, and you were allowed to have one when your turn came in the queue. The water came from a rigged-up garden hose thrown over the side of a sloping mud wall. Propped up against this was a shower cubicle, a dark thatched lean-to about the size of a telephone box and, after hanging your towel outside, into the murky depths you plunged.

Thirty seconds after going in, you emerged into the sunlight again either scalded or shivering, depending on your place in the queue. You then quickly rushed your clothes back on before anything else could have a go at you. That night in bed you came across the bumps and itches where the shower's permanent inhabitants had had their revenge.

But help was on the way in the form of a new boarding school 150 miles away, near the township of Iringa. It was called St Michael's and St George's and next term we were all going there. It had proper buildings made of brick, inside loos, large bathrooms with washbasins and showers, an assembly hall – and proper teachers flown out from the UK. There was also a proper headmaster, depending on how you define these things. He wore a black mortar board and gown, and carried a long, swishing cane. He thought black people and teenagers needed plenty of discipline and punishment.

Iringa, like Kongwa, was co-educational, so we were acclimatised to boys and didn't get hysterical and distracted from our work at the sight of one. But our own bodies were a different matter. With comfortable surroundings at our disposal, self-awareness arrived like a plague. What to do with it, though, when you lived in a school with no mirrors?

The Head was a puritan. Looking at ourselves would be bad for our personalities, he said, and he only allowed small mirrors on the inside of our locker doors – enough to see the middle bit of a face in, just about.

So, lady-dom in Africa was a co-operative enterprise. We managed our mirror-less days by looking out for each other:

'Is my petticoat showing at the back?' 'Can you see my bra strap through this?' 'Does this make my hips look big?' 'Is my hair sticking out?'

We stood by too: seeing a girl's petticoat showing as we said prayers before mealtimes, or her collar turned up at the back, was reason to risk extra prep by whispering the news across the table and down the opposite line.

Sex wasn't the reason we were keeping ourselves up-to-scratch, at least not that we dared admit, as the rumours were sobering. Someone said once you did it you were a slave to it and wanted it all the time and didn't think about anything else and couldn't do your work. 'Ooh,' we groaned in despair.

Then there was the one about once you did it, you'd be found out because of something that happened to your eyes, a change of some kind. 'Ooh,' we groaned again.

There were other kinds of rumours: some still imagined babies came out, Caesarian-style, through our stomachs; others thought menstrual blood caused warts; and Veronica thought 'hymen' was a Latin verb. Anna was convinced the hymen was at the back of your throat and would be broken through French kissing, which she therefore viewed as disgusting. A lot of us didn't know what French kissing was, but would rather die than say so.

With smokescreens, shock tactics, oohings and aahings, we fought off desire as best we could. But it was in us and, knowing no other way, we attacked it. Pain was the method, hair the target and 'off with it' the chorus. A pubic strand escaping the swimsuit line, fuzzy down on the side of a cheek, hair round a nipple, a shadow circling a navel, all of it was attacked with the fervour my boyhood self had kept for a different kind of natural world.

Boys smacked the nature outside of themselves. It seems girls had to smack the nature *inside*.

Around this time, I experienced my first brief glimpse of the claustrophobia which was to trouble me fifteen years later in London lifts and tubes.

Getting bold by now, one quiet Saturday afternoon, Linde, who slept next to me, decided to lead an expeditionary force from our dorm to visit the boys. Since the boys' dorms were out of bounds on threat of expulsion, Linde hit on the idea of crawling through a network of unused water pipes which ran from

Pritchard House, where we slept, all the way to the boys' dorms at the other end of the school.

The concrete pipes were broad enough for a body to crawl through, so after a few hours of dolling ourselves up – plucking, shaving legs, showering, combing, tweaking and checking each other over for odd bits sticking out anywhere – we put on our most revealing shorts and set off.

Linde was in the lead, and I was bringing up the rear, until, that is, about fifty yards in, when a first awareness of panic at how enclosed I was caught me and I knew I had to get out fast, while I could.

'I'm going back,' I said, my voice booming through the concrete chamber.

The fear was fleeting, gone as soon as I emerged from the pipeline, and I dismissed it from my mind. It didn't stop me spending hours in other confined places. Mock O levels were looming, and we searched determinedly for places to study. 'Lights out' was prompt at 9 p.m., and we needed more time to cram. There were lights in the loos so we made up an occupying force. With four cubicles – one girl sitting on the loo and another wedged against the door – eight girls could swot for an hour then wake up the next eight. We did fine for a week or so. Then Biddy, our House mistress, got wind of us.

A few nights later, we hit on the linen cupboard. This took six girls at a time under the same system of waking up the next six on your way back to bed. But then Biddy came looking for some spare bedding.

But before sitting the exams, which I was taking a year early, trouble with my eyes started: not lack of sleep, but hockey. We played on a red earth pitch, dust storms blowing at regular intervals and my large eyes, acting as dustbins, got redder and redder. Whingeing to Biddy was no good. She told me straight: if I stayed out of lavatories and linen cupboards at night and went to bed instead, my eyes would be better in no time.

Soon after a specialist in Nairobi diagnosed trachoma which could cause blindness, and advised an immediate trip back to the UK, to Moorfields eye hospital. There was a branch of Moorfields outside Croydon in Surrey, only a few miles away from Nellie.

Chapter Nineteen

❧

NELLIE'S WRATH . . . AND CHILDHOOD

Nellie was the woman my father went to war for and she was in and out of my childhood, affecting what I did, even from thousands of miles away. When she stayed with us, on the RAF base when I was six, there was some protection from her growing dislike of me. But being with her on my own, I felt the full force of her violent feelings towards me – and her wish to change the very nature of my bones.

A few days after my arrival in Surrey, Nellie brought in a burly woman in a tweed suit, a friend of hers and a neighbour. Hand-picked for the task, this woman made it clear that if I gave my grandmother any trouble at all I would have to live with *her*. If that happened, I would be locked in my room as soon as I came home from school, my mail would be vetted, and I would live alone.

I plummeted. As a teenager in Africa, I'd grown used to bright sunlight, a swimming pool, diving, a big sky, dancing, playing tennis, being out most of the time. Now, I was threatened with being a prisoner. I kept out of Nellie's way, retreating upstairs to my bedroom where she couldn't get me.

By day I went to a comprehensive school in Warlingham, having failed to get into the smart girls' grammar nearby. Just as well. I had few suitable clothes with me for meeting people after school. What with her age and her false leg, Nellie couldn't help me shop for an English winter and I had little money of my own.

Circumstances bleak, I gained weight, grew spots, and rued the treatments from Moorfields which made my eyes sticky.

Although the complaint turned out not to be trachoma, it took eight long months to get my eyes somewhere near right again. A form of acute – and chronic – conjunctivitis was diagnosed, needing extensive treatment. Nellie must have been coming up to her seventieth year, too old to cook and care for any grandchild, let alone one who produced in her the feelings I did.

Escaping from the house to walk, sometimes, along the Godstone road into Purley, I longed for someone to recognise me, fantasised about hearing the magic word: 'Carol' shouted from a passing car. I dreamed that someone from Africa or Wales would be on the road, spot me – and make everything all right again. For I didn't feel myself. The sad, podgy, bleary-eyed girl I had become wasn't really me.

When a tall Australian boy called Andrew asked me out on the school stairway one day, shouting my name from the floor above, I thought I had been recognised at last. The son of a visiting diplomat, his family lived in a big, beautiful house, and he invited me to meet them for Sunday tea. But Nellie insisted I wear my school uniform. My hard-fought-for compromise, half uniform and half not, looked a mess. Ill at ease, I wasn't asked back.

Away from Nellie, in my bedroom upstairs, I wrote my poems. I'd written hundreds and collected them into about a dozen hard-backed exercise books. My precious cargo, I kept them close to me. They said more about me than anything or anyone else. In boarding school in Tanzania, they were kept next to my bed. Now, in Purley, they were in the same place, near me in the dark.

But the lure of TV brought me down sometimes to sit in awkward silence, Nellie in one chair, me in the other. One night she could bear it no longer:

'You're just like your mother,' she flung at me. 'You're the spitting image of her, and your mother ruined my son's life. She brought him down in the world with her flighty ways, her and her lipstick and . . .'

Nellie's rant was awful to watch as well as hear. She sneered and mocked my mother: her hair, clothes, her way of holding her head high. That Nellie hated my mother I'd glimpsed, but that anyone could deride her like this, I couldn't bear.

'How dare you say that about my mother.' I shouted.

'It's no use defending her,' Nellie came back. 'You're tarred with the same brush. You'll get into trouble, you will.'

'No I won't. She's much nicer than you. You shouldn't say these things.'

My mother being my first soft spot, Nellie then hit the second.

'You think you can hide those silly poems. Well, when you're at school I'm going to go into your bedroom and look at them.'

Out of my chair I jumped:

'I'll burn them first. I'll burn them before letting you see them.'

'Go on, then,' said Nellie.

By the time I came down the stairs with what I loved most clasped tight to my chest, Nellie had the matches in her hands.

The tiny back garden was behind the kitchen, and Nellie stomped round the blaze the poems made as they went up in flames in the crisp winter's night. I can't say for sure she chuckled and incanted, but she seemed like a witch to me that night, and that is how I viewed her for the rest of her life.

She was eighty-seven when she died. I was working for a TV company in London and could have gone to her funeral. But staying with my English grandmother had stripped me of love. I went to Paris for the weekend instead. Years later, a story her daughter, my aunt, told me by a Maidstone hearth made me relent. But how to begin?

My grandmother was a hunchback – a problem with her bones, especially her spine. Before that, even, there was a stigma, a thwarted love affair and a tragedy. A Welshman, a Mr Hughes, robbed her of her first – and only – chance of ease. He stole a garden from her, and changed the shape of her life. Tied up in the conventions of Victorian Middle England, the knot which kept this story secret lasted 100 years and damaged many people's lives.

Nellie was born out of wedlock to a middle-class mother, Grace, who got pregnant by her sister's husband. In fact Grace and the man had been unofficially engaged, but her socially aspiring parents wanted to marry off their elder daughter, Flo, first. It was the proper thing to do in the kind of middle to upper middle-class circles they were moving in.

So, this marriage of convenience was forced on everyone, but the natural lovers met after the wedding, Grace continuing a relationship with her older sister's new husband – and my grandmother was the result. Some months before Nellie was born, Grace was thrown out of the comfortable home she shared with her parents when they learned she was pregnant.

It was the winter of 1888. It was cold, conditions were harsh and for that year, and for many years that followed, Nellie's mother could barely feed herself let alone her child. Nellie developed rickets soon after her eighth birthday. The hump on her back was the result of this lack of calcium and rose like a pyramid from her right shoulder. Although Nellie was not a *Nôtre Dame*-type hunchback, for she was tall, this piece of bleak bonework made her shoulder and the upper half of her body stooped and mis-shapen, which is how it remained till she died.

She also had a curvature in her spine, which wasn't helped by the heavy bundles she carried to and from train stations as a child in the 1890s. She brought sewing to the factories, work her mother took on to get money to feed them both, Nellie acting as courier. Nellie was afraid, on these journeys, of the money she collected being stolen from her. Pressing herself into the seat, wanting to be invisible, she stared hard through the window.

Before Nellie was nine, her mother met and married a Mr Wellard, and had two more girls, Gladys and Margaret. But then Mr Wellard quit the family, leaving them all penniless once more.

Flo and her husband had come up in the world, having connections with Edward the VII himself. Nellie's father was one of the King's sporting companions and her cousin was presented at court.

They were now in a position to make a gift, to buy Nellie's mother and her three girls a large property with a big walled garden in Hanover Park, Peckham, South London. There the family would be self-sufficient by taking in respectable gentleman lodgers and tending an already beautiful garden. The first of these 'gentlemen' was Mr Hughes.

Nellie was twelve years old when Mr Hughes and her mother set up home together as man and wife. Life was going to be good now. At last. No more struggling with bundles of sewing, no more hunger, or living in two rooms. There would be no more rough glances from men on trains or fear of being robbed on the way home. Nellie would spend her time planting and tending flowers in a place where things were safe.

Then, one evening, Mr Hughes gave Grace the news which Nellie never recovered from – her elder daughter would have to go:

'I'll take on them,' he said about Maggic and Gladys, 'but not the hunchback' – and Grace gave her daughter away. Nellie was sent into service, to get up at 5 a.m. and clean grates. Through tenacity, intelligence and sheer guts, she worked her way up from the bottom grate to learning how to cook, and by the time she was twenty-six she was assistant cook to a large family in Bexhill-on-Sea.

At a local Salvation Army meeting she met Owen Lee, a man who was sickly when she married him, and who remained that way all his life.

He had pernicious anaemia, which was to kill him eventually, but there was no diagnosis for it at that time and he was labelled a malingerer. Both the illness itself and the mocking names he was called in the village because he didn't work meant Owen spent most of his time sitting in a corner, deeply depressed. His wife and children were ridiculed because of him, and life was hard for them all.

During the 1920s, as times got even harder and jobs more scarce, Welshmen crossed the border to take the jobs Owen Lee couldn't hold down. The Welsh miners were desperate and some of them left their homes to work in England for less money than their English counterparts. Nellie raged against this, as she raged about anything connected with Wales.

Nellie hated my mother for being Welsh and for trapping her only son into marriage. My arrival, less than five months after the wedding, she blamed on my mother and myself. My aunt describes an incident from my childhood when I brought back some stowaways from a holiday in Wales. It was during the Sanderstead days when I was around four, and hiding in my thick ringlets were dozens of *Welsh* head-lice. They were further proof for Nellie that the whole of Wales was one huge crawling tip of dirt and depravity.

'People are filthy down there,' she spat at her daughter while my mother was within hearing. Then, out it came, about Welsh people keeping coal in the bath, and living in caves and not going to church. My mother heard it all. The three of us, Nellie, my mother and myself, had to go to the local fumigation department to be seen to, me the only one with a smile on my face.

So, this was my grandmother. She hated my Welsh

mother and my mother felt all this and began to lose her hair.

Even when Nellie was ill and lived with us while my mother nursed her, there was a 'coal-hole' inside her, a black place which she couldn't keep a lid on. She would tell me, when I was alone, that my mother thought I was a horrible little girl. She would then tell my mother, when I was not in the room, that I had cheeked her; she would tell my father, when neither of us was around, that his family was getting out of control and he had better put his foot down. She would then watch as we acted out the parts she had set us up for.

My father never spotted this. His mother being tricky with people was how she was. She was hectoring with the men her daughters married too.

I was in my late teens before I saw what she did. It was usually a late morning start, shortly before lunch when she stoked us all up. After she watched us have a tense meal, she would go to bed for her daily nap. She would wake up from this sleep sweet-tempered and smiling. The rest of us at it hammer and tongs, Nellie would watch the drama, smiling as she sat in her chair. It was her late afternoon theatre.

How did she get away with it? As with my father, God was on her side. She was a pillar of the local church, a bible-reading, God-fearing woman – and my mother couldn't fight that. Not until long after Nellie died could my father accept the damage his mother did.

But then, in her own life as a parent, Nellie collapsed

a number of times from nervous exhaustion, or mood swings. She was taken away to be looked after, sometimes by nuns, in a deathly-quiet equivalent of a mental ward. While she was gone, her two daughters were thought able to manage for themselves, but the youngest child, my father, was put to an orphanage.

'The place was cruel', my aunt recalled. 'It was terribly sad, how badly the children were treated. They were hit for the least thing, kept cold and hungry and only occasionally allowed out for a visit. It was an awful, bleak place.'

On one of his occasional visits to see his mother, longing as a small boy to be with her again, my father thought the silent nuns with their winged cowls and rustling clothes were angels, and his mother dead. She lay like a corpse. Still and white against the sheets, as she would be when her leg was blown off a decade or more later, my father longed for her return to life.

With her family at mealtimes there was, as well, Nellie's hunger. Sometimes she eked out food and there was none left for herself. Plate empty, she sat with them, head bowed, hands clasped together in her lap.

I knew nothing of this till my incapacity caused me to spend weekends by my aunt's hearth, and the story of Nellie's life fell into my lap.

An ability to float out of your body as a six-year-old child in a car and, later, as a fifteen-year-old returning to

Africa, can probably not be called up unless there is good reason to find and use it hard. Nellie was such a reason. The cutting edge of her tongue, and the X-ray shaming of her eyes, increased with the years as I came to be less of a child and more of a woman, with much of my mother in me.

It's possible she hated my mother, not only for being Welsh, but for being extrovert and pretty, for having a straight, supple body, and for being a beautiful dancer. But in pictures taken when she was younger, when she had long, thick hair, Nellie herself looks lovely. She has beautiful skin, large grey-blue eyes and is beguilingly wistful. She loved the stage, and was a good mimic and actress. Her daughter remembers her playing the role of a town crier at a summer fete, her strange shape silhouetted against a marquee on a Surrey village green.

She also remembers Nellie finding herself a second 'husband'. Only a year or two after Owen's death, Nellie went round the corner from her Purley home to catch a bus. Stomping along to the end of the bus queue in her ungainly way, without knowing it, she trod hard on a man's foot.

Bristling at her unconcern, Arthur Santer tapped her on the shoulder:

'Madam, don't you usually apologise when you break someone's toe?'

Nellie took one look at his blue eyes and handsome face framed by a mane of white hair, and batted her eyelids hard:

'Oh dear' she sighed, in one of her best sing-song modes. 'It must have been my wooden one.'

They didn't get married, Arthur Santer and herself, but they lived as close companions: shopping together; travelling to see family and friends; an inseparable pair. Standing in the doorway in her dressing gown, Nellie saw off the vicar when he called round one Saturday morning to 'have a talk about her circumstances'.

When 'Pop Santa', as I called him, died more than ten years ahead of her, Nellie took herself off to a Methodist retirement home so as not to be a burden to any of her children; the truth being none of them could have lived with her. I last saw her a few years before her death, and she was tricky with me then too, so I left her be.

Chapter Twenty

᪥

AN ELEPHANT IN THE GARDEN

Returning to East Africa after living with Nellie, setting fire to my poems may have robbed me of more than words – and made me vulnerable to what followed.

Back in boarding school at the age of fifteen, with only a few months left to swot for GCSEs, I was welcomed back on the night shift as if I'd never been gone. But by day something odd was happening: a peculiar feeling of remoteness; like being an island surrounded by sea and cut off from activity around me. Then headaches, feeling faint, a loss of appetite. Biddy did not, of course, believe me. It wasn't until my temperature hit 104° that she got out her red MG and raced me to the sickbay.

Most grown-ups are unfathomable when you're fifteen, their behaviour as bizarre to you as yours is to them. But I really thought Sister was off her trolley when, as I slowly lapsed into unconsciousness, she kept on shaking me to ask in her hard German accent: 'Where do you come from, child. Where do you live?' I didn't understand the questions. I had come from Pritchard House, with Biddy there to prove it, but it must have got through to me she was asking where my home was. So I mumbled 'Mwadui' before passing out. A cursory glance at a map in those days showed Mwadui as a cerebral malaria zone, and that is what I had.

I was 'gone' for a week, the relevance of where I lived, or anything else, lost on me. But was I unconscious? From all I remember, I spent the week on the ceiling. Hovering above a single bed, I looked down on the small isolation room with its west-facing window where people worked hard on an inert figure – my body. Sometimes they swaddled it with blankets and hot water bottles. At other times, they covered it with cold towels dipped in buckets full of cold water and ice.

Feeling nothing, I watched this work continuing on the figure in the bed. Then one evening I woke up, integrated again: weak, but in one piece. Lying still, I watched the light fade and long shadows arrive. Listening to trees rustling outside and the returning sounds of African voices, I knew I was back.

The physical part of my illness was the fever, but I believe the floating part was Nellie. As a six-year-old, rubbing my forefinger and thumb together in the back seat of my father's car, I had summoned up the earth against her, drifting away on a round globe as big as the world.

Growing up, I too easily believed people who didn't like me could 'put me out', turn off the light in me, which is what I feared Nellie would do. And there was something I had to save.

In the term before going to stay with Nellie, a poem was 'dictated' to me in the night. Woken by a figure or voice in my head, I was led through sleeping bodies in the dormitory, down the steps, out into the hall and round the corner to where long glass doors locked us in for the night. There, by starlight, I obeyed this ghost or angel in my head – and wrote down what it told me.

I had to save this – and my other poems – from Nellie's prying eyes. But in switching them off, had I rescued or lost them? New poems would grow years later, after Nellie's death, but for now, down from the ceiling, there was silence inside me. I'd killed the story of my life and already there were so many deaths and killings.

I sat GCSEs in a dream.

Arriving in Mwadui for the school holidays, I heard my mother one day, try to get my father concerned about my continuing thinness from the fever:

'She's like a skeleton. You can see all her ribs.'

But my father showed no interest in my near-death from cerebral malaria. There were bad rows between us by this time. I had to accept his God before my father would accept me – and I wouldn't. With a growing command of language, I threw my words, fistfuls of them, at my father, resisting him and his God, refusing to go to the church where He lived.

Churches made me miserable. They stole from me, took my joy. Going in one robbed me of hope, strength, vitality.

'Your God hates children,' I shouted. 'I won't have anything to do with Him. You can do what you like. You can starve me if you want. I don't care.'

During these rows my mother was angry with us both and, if she couldn't stop us, left us to it and went next door. My brother Chris, as a four-year-old, stood by, taking my part:

'You mustn't do that to Carol,' he yelled. 'Stoppit.'

As a boy child, whom my father could more easily accept and understand, he was listened to, and when he raced in between us, hitting my father's legs with his fists, shouting at him to leave me alone, my father would tousle the top of his head, and let me be.

What I feared most during the rows was bursting into tears – a sign of weakness – and if this was coming on, I ran to my bedroom. A soft knock on the door, and my brother's voice. Sometimes I told him to go away, and sometimes I let him come in and sit with me. He put his hand in mine or stroked my arm:

'Don't cry,' he'd say. 'I'll make you better.'

But once my angry words were done, there was guilt and despair in place of relief or triumph, a corner of me still wanting my father to love me. But the rows sent us further apart. I stayed out – away from my father – and from his.

Animals were my refuge. Only a short distance from

the high security wire fence which was Mwadui's boundary, the African plains were almost unchanged: flocks of flamingo, herds of elephant, giraffe, rhino, leopard, impala, gazelle, zebra, wildebeast, buffalo, vividly coloured bee-eaters, rollers, owls. Standing by a baobab tree one day, on an illicit expedition into the bush, elephant were standing nearby: a large family group, young ones playing unthreatened, the elders peaceful. There was none of the torment and despair of my own life in theirs. Things were as they should be with the animals.

Inside the fence in Mwadui were the sunshine, rock 'n' rolling, playing with my brother and diving into the swimming pool days which were the envy of my school mates. While other settlers had a hard time, often just a few families living together with no running water or electricity, we had comfort – and luxury even. There were proper houses, running water, a golf course, swimming pool, tennis courts, cinema, club house and a fleet of Dakotas to fly in fresh food from Nairobi.

I relished Mwadui: luxury inside the gates, and outside bush to explore, animals to see, space, air, a sense of timelessness – freedom. Unbeknown to my parents, a friend's father, Old Man Kennedy, used to loan us his Land Rover for the day. A diamond prospector working in the scrubland, the deal was we drove him to his patch first and picked him up before sundown.

We were about a dozen teenagers in the settlement –

some 150 or so European families – and we gathered in the evenings at the club house where our parents drank and held open-air dances. One night we formed a circle slightly away from the lights of the club on a piece of open ground. The night sounds and the dark formed a curtain between us and the watching eyes and ears of the adults.

We put on some favourite music – Kwela – a breathy, tin-whistle sound on top, and underneath a steady, hypnotic beat. In and out of the notes we danced, jumping up and down like acrobats in the dark – straight into a trance. When the whistle slowly wound down, we returned, twitching awake one at a time, breaking the spell. Our bodies heavy, we were deep-eyed with the need to sleep.

In the daytime, sitting at home with my brother while our mother shopped at the duka, there was once a marvellous visitor came to see us. I was sat on the steps reading in the shade of the wide verandah round our bungalow. A bush garden with trees, shrubs, and a high, thick hedge shielded us from the dirt road beyond.

My brother played happily in these afternoons, in and out of bushes, picking up insects, chasing lizards, catching chameleons, tracing trails with his finger in the red earth. He was playing, me glancing up from time to time to make sure he wasn't on the road, when I saw something approaching along the other side of the hedge. An elephant trunk is what it looked like, but it was not until the creature came round the corner that I fully believed my eyes. There it stood, on our gravel path, young and lost, but still huge compared to us and, as it happened, hopeful. It wanted to be friends.

It was about a year old and eager to make contact. When my brother, who was four, squealed and ran towards it, they greeted each other like old friends. I watched for a while as they played together, my brother so small and the elephant taller than I was.

Then I remembered my manners and fetched the garden hose. Our visitor probably needed a drink. But at the sound of water in the pipe coils, it came charging towards me and, as the first trickle came out, nearly devoured the hose. Squashed up against the wall of the house, I tried to wrest the hose away, but the elephant was winning. It had me pinned and I was gasping for breath.

'Quick, turn off the tap,' I shouted to my brother.

It was his chance to get rid of a bossy older sister – but he did as I asked.

Getting round the animal's eagerness, we filled buckets of water at the garden tap and, when its thirst was quenched, sprayed the hose over its body. Then it had a play. Half a ton of undiluted, unselfconscious cavorting delight, it danced in the sun, and the more we laughed, the more it performed exuberant tricks. Round it twirled, running in one direction at full speed and then turning and racing off in another, then twirling round and round again. It flung back its trunk, flapped its ears, trumpeted in a rather squeaky, juvenile way and showered us with spray. All the while it was careful of the small boy racing under its body and trying to swing on its trunk.

Our garden friend stayed late, only trotting away in a deep huff after an encounter with my mother's still-zealous housekeeping habits. She polished everything she could lay her duster on, including the verandah steps. When I went in for a drink, it tried to follow me up and found its large padded feet acting like rotating electric polishers on the highly shone surface. Alarmed at having its front legs taken from under it by some demon verandah magic, off it went.

These holiday times of orphaned elephant and roaming deer, of black mambas curled up in settee springs and my brother and I collapsing with laughter when my mother shrieked, and lizards climbing curtain rails, of swimming-pool days and dancing nights, of lazy verandah reading times and drives in the bush, then ended.

The late loo-sitting, cupboard-occupying and solidarity of the night shift at Iringa had got me the equivalent of eight O levels – and I was to fly back to Wales to Harry and Bessie for further schooling. The thinking was this: big changes were afoot in East Africa. Independence – Uhuru – already granted, and Tanganyika changing to Tanzania, you couldn't be sure the Iringa teachers – all employed straight from the UK – would renew their contracts to see me through A levels. So, I would leave.

There was no way, now, of saying goodbye to anyone at Iringa. We were scattered round thousands of miles in the school holidays. But then 'goodbye' was never my favourite word. I didn't know, daren't know, what it meant. For I had been apart from and with my parents for much of my life, on a string or a thread. They were there and not. 'Goodbye' wasn't spoken. 'Cheerio for now' was my father's way – and my mother's? Withdrawal. Whether to ease a child's pain or her own wasn't clear. Neither was it clear, as now, if I would ever be back.

I was content to go, oddly enough, for East Africa had rebuilt my confidence and I was planning for something it couldn't give me – a place at a British university. I felt sure if I worked hard, I would get one. The future beckoned once more: big, warm and as captivating and full of life as the country I was leaving.

Chapter Twenty-One

⋙

PROCRUSTES SITS

It's a phrase of Renzo's I come back to: 'I can work on the muscles. Only you can work on the mind.' As if my part of it's simple, like the click of a spine. As if a woman with God in her ribcage can be free in an instant. I resent him his easier task.

He's trying to prise apart the steel bands I've constructed from the muscles around my thorax, my suit of armour. Using his version of a technique called 'inhibition', instead of countering the strain, he goes with it first.

Renzo explains that if you take something which is very tense and try to pull it, it will snap back into its original position, or be weakened by being pulled away from what it's used to. If you relax the muscle first, it will reposition itself 'with more confidence'.

I've been wearing my steel breastplate since childhood

to defend myself against the hurt of Nellie, God and my father. I shored myself up against them and many times faced 'death' in the sense of knowing I'd rather die than be their creature. They wanted to deform me, make me other than who I was. So it was war and I didn't know my limits in fending off these tyrants. But it wasn't only war. It was sunlight too – and laughter, the parts of me that had nothing to do with them. My life was extreme: filled with danger, then soft African mornings; captivity, then startling escapes – out of a box, on to a ceiling.

My return to Wales at the age of sixteen gives a glimpse of these two extremes: fight and flight; sunshine and darkness; and of the schizophrenic nature of an inner world where I plunged between them, as if I lived on the inside in two separate places, two different rooms.

The sunshine side of my life was African freedom, the open air, vast skies – and a young elephant in the garden. It was sitting on the floor of a Tanzanian bungalow, bribing my brother with sweets to brush my long hair till it shone and his arm ached. It was him hiding his small brother's offerings of dead insects and creatures in my bedroom when I was in the shower, then leaving one of his toys on the floor as a 'Watch out, I've been about' calling card. It was me screeching when I tripped over his token of half a bat, a few spiders or some assorted scorpions. Then, clutching a towel round myself, chasing him along the hallway, into the garden, round and round the house, through the hedge into the garden next door, and eventually catching him because he was laughing so much he fell helpless to the ground.

It was watching rhino at dawn in a landscape almost unchanged in tens of thousands of years – the feeling this was the first day in the world and I was in it. How could a girl with this much Africa in her be afraid? But I was.

The fearful other place inside me was a dark room where I inhabited a mass of nameless, faceless guilt and anxiety, a ghost train ride of tendrils across my face and lurchings in my stomach. In this room I was blind, or else it was so black I couldn't see, and blindness was foisted on me. I lost sight of myself, of my hands, my feet, my heart. For, in truth, this was a heartless place. My 'badness' in this room was everything, and as palpable as a young elephant in the other.

There was something else too. In the dark place, a shadowy male figure had charge of my oxygen supply as I lay, desperately ill, in a hospital bed – or sometimes my own. At times a giant figure and at others human-sized, it was only his shape I saw, his back hunched, on occasion, as he leaned forward, sometimes by my side, at others from behind my head. Like Nellie, he could snuff me out at the flick of a finger or the turn of a switch. But why?

What I was guilty of I didn't know. It was as if I had broken something once, and my family had been a happy place, me safe within it, until I did this. Whatever I had broken had happened when I was small, because

I didn't remember a time *before* 'broken'.

Sometimes I felt I could mend it, whatever it was, because in a normal forgiving world you can do that. You can have a second chance, especially if you didn't break it on purpose. In the dark room I knew I couldn't mend it because once something is cracked it can never be the same again.

Too late has already happened.

In Wales Harry and Bessie's house was still full. Before my arrival my uncles were turfed out of their beds and my cousin Derek sent to lodgings at the other end of the village so I could have a bedroom to myself. I returned to find him working as an apprentice roofer staying with his boss and family, and I wasn't told the reason why. So, three people were out of their beds, and no one was happy except, perhaps, Bessie, who liked having a girl around. But I appeared to be an ungrateful one. I was still squeamish about dirty towels and a bar of soap with black grit in it from the mines, though I tried to hide it.

I didn't see Derek except on the odd Sunday when he came for food and our eyes slid off each other's like the marbles we played with as children.

Attending Gwendraeth Grammar School with all this inside me, I was snapped up by the drama master for a part in the school's production of *Lady Windermere's Fan*. It was the 'light and shade' in my voice he was after, he said, its 'emotional range'. I enjoyed rehearsals, being up onstage, where the staff stood for assembly, and throwing my voice out to the back of the hall. But I wasn't there the night of the performance. After some weeks of rehearsals I had to back out, for there was nowhere in 77 for me to learn the lines.

The downstairs was cluttered with uncles, neighbours, second cousins, neighbours' children vying to be Harry's favourite, and Bessie doing Welsh songs and Chopin waltzes on the piano. She had formed a dance band by this time, The Montana Melody Makers. An eight-piece ensemble, it provided money and gave her a way of playing music. Her being the leader of the band, you sometimes got people dropping in for bookings or practice.

Then there were Harry's activities: ludo, card-playing and telling stories. You couldn't learn lines of your own in the middle of Harry's stories. And, in any case, if there were any theatricals going on in the house, he was in charge – and he'd never heard of *Lady Windermere's Fan*.

It was winter. Upstairs was freezing – and there was the disappearing light bulb. Downstairs there were two – in the front room where the piano was, and the scullery where we ate food – so you couldn't borrow one. Upstairs there was one in the middle of my bedroom ceiling, and it vanished – I suspect into my uncle Alan's pocket. Something told me it would be better not to ask for it back.

The other thing you had to do was guard your flannel with your life. If you left it undefended in the bathroom for even a minute it would disappear like a light bulb.

This environment was where I tried to study with the idea of earning myself a place at university.

'Carol, who was Procrustes?' the English teacher asked one day as he read passages of text aloud. I had no idea and, skirting back for clues in the just-spoken lines, saw only the word 'Procrustean' flashing at me. After a long pause, I had to say:

'I don't know, sir.'

There were only four of us for A level English: two boys, Brian and Arwel; and two girls, Margaret and myself – the youngest. So you couldn't hide. Turning to this small group, his voice laden with sarcasm, the teacher said:

'This girl just hasn't been educated, has she?'

I was mortified. Still a relative stranger in the class, English, which was my best subject, began to be a nightmare. My body played up in class and I could do nothing to stop it. However full or empty it was, my stomach would set up a din like the rumblings of a herd of elephants. I began to feel sick, and to have headaches and to long, every moment of the lessons, for them to end.

It's lodged in my mind who Procrustes was – a fabled Greek innkeeper, alias robber, who kept only one size of bed at his thieving establishment. When guests/victims came to stay, he chopped inches off them or stretched them to fit this bed size. 'Procrustean' means violently changing or adapting the wrong element of something to make it conform to a standard – like the English master did to children. His reputation for being stern and unyielding in pursuit of educational ideals was known throughout the school.

Another time, he asked me if I did my homework in the middle of my dinner because it had stains on it. In fact, I did my homework, when I could, in the middle of dollops of gravy, vinegar, jam, mint sauce, custard, tea and runny rice pudding. Your chances of hitting a dry patch on the dark floral oilcloth on our kitchen table were slight. A dishcloth in the house made occasional appearances, but you could never rely on it. It was probably somebody's ex-flannel and led a wraith-like existence. I spotted it coming out of Bessie's pinafore pocket once or twice, but then it was gone again.

Had he been a different kind of person, I might have confided in the English master that I was having problems, but I couldn't imagine saying: 'I'm sorry I haven't done the essay, sir, but there were lots of things happening in our house last night. Glynn was doing trumpet practice, and then people came into the front room to sing songs. I would have gone in the scullery, but my grandfather was playing ludo with Mr Rumbelow, and they were shouting and arguing a lot, like they usually do. Then the electricity went out, and we didn't have a shilling for the meter, and we spent half an hour looking for where my grandmother had put the candles . . .'

My grandmother, not thinking to put candles in the same place twice, never practised lifting a duster, darning a sock or boiling an egg either. When making a Sunday lunch she put the cabbage on at the same time as the meat and sat down to play music. Three or four hours later, the greens were swimming in an evil smelling swamp which she then cheerfully advised you to drink. Good for the complexion, she said.
I decided I preferred having spots.

But I was beguiled by Harry and Bessie, the activity in the house; people calling to ask my grandmother to play or to listen to another of Harry's silver-tongued stories.

I was swayed in another way as well. Harry thought too much homework and reading was bad for your personality, especially if you were a girl. He thought you were supposed to live your life, not bury yourself in books, and he had something else on his wily mind which led to some spats between us.

'What's the point of all those books when you're only going to get married?' he'd say to me. 'What use'll they be to you then?'

'I'm not going to get married. I'm going to go to university and have a good job and a career.'

'That's what you think. You watch out. There'll be a rich farmer will catch you. Then it will be up at five with the cows . . .'

'I'm not listening to you.' I'd be shouting by then. 'You wait and see. I'm never, ever, going to marry a farmer.'

'Well, you'd better learn to run then,' he'd round off with a twinkle. 'One's bound to catch you if you don't.'

Rows with Harry were never bad affairs.

Bessie, too, took an active interest in my boyfriends but she knew what Harry wouldn't see, that I was too young, yet, to think of settling. It was she who encouraged me, then, to play the field.

Who was I going out with this week? she would ask. Was I still seeing so-and-so? No? Well I was young. Plenty of time.

One night, in that first summer in Wales, when I was still sixteen, I went to a dance with a crowd of older girls from the village. We were supposed to come straight home afterwards. Instead, the others decided to go to the beach in a big crowd of much older people I had never met. Not wanting to be a spoilsport, I said nothing.

Sitting for a while, by myself in the dark, I listened to murmurings around me, laughter as people drifted up the beach together. Suddenly my heart started pounding. The people I had come with melted into the darkness, I thought I would never find my way back to Harry and Bessie again. I was lost. The return of an old terror: being engulfed by the dark; of it being never-ending; of losing myself in it and having the people I cared for disappear.

What was disappearing in my life was my future, the prospect of a place at university: three years in one place to make friends; to be part of a group of people my own age; to study, talk, laugh, debate; to make up for the moves and chaos of the past.

Trying to do homework, I'd borrowed a neighbour's front room when it was free, but she was part of the 'front parlour is only for special occasions' brigade. About once every three weeks seemed to be the parlour's tolerance for company, and it wasn't enough.

Slowly, shamefacedly, I slid backwards at school. Mumbling excuses about the essays I hadn't done, I avoided teachers' eyes. Instead of schoolwork, I began to write things I already knew and could work on in the corner with noise all round. Stories. About Africa mainly.

Africa was another one of the things that had gone away from me and which I wanted to keep. Africa inside me meant the ability to be confident and strong. Unlike my last time in Wales when I was ten, I knew Africa wasn't a dream, but I wasn't sure about *myself*. In Mwadui I had been certain of my life. Now it was sliding from me. I'd lost it again.

Struggling, I wondered had the real me stayed behind in Africa or was the real me here? We were different. There was the person who wasn't afraid of an elephant and the one who was afraid of the dark. Was there more than one of me? And, if there was, how could I get the other one back? And was that the right thing to do?

Chapter Twenty-Two

THE SUIT

Renzo is annoying me again. He says, in his cheerful way, that my exaggerated S-bending spine has made me develop a 'wrong' posture which has thrown me out of true. I argue:

'I've spent a lifetime standing up straight.'

'No, no,' he says. 'When you say you are standing up straight, you are leaning a lot forwards. Look.'

That spring, in Wales, I had many fantasies about moving forwards, of being an independent woman with a job and a home of my own where there was quiet to read – and peace to write. I sometimes saw this woman I was to become, beckoning me, urging me on. Always the same age – twenty-five – I saw her in my dreams at night and in odd glances in the mirror by day. She was tall, calm and confident and seemed to say to me that if I would go with her, life would be all right at last, that too late hadn't already happened, that the future was a big place with room for me to be happy. At sixteen, I wanted to believe I hadn't lost all my chances already, for however I struggled, the prospect of a university place had gone from being near and attainable to beyond my reach.

The weather helped with the plan which came to mind when I went to bed one night. That was the year there wasn't a sunny day between May and September, so I didn't mind being stuck indoors. At half term, I got up early one morning and set off. I was going to go out and find myself a job, any job, for the summer holidays. I knew I couldn't leave school yet because I was still only sixteen, and probably no one would let me. I wasn't sure if anyone made decisions about me any more, but I could start saving money for when I was ready to have a life of my own.

In heavy rain, I hitched a lift some seventy miles to Tenby. There, I looked for a street where there were plenty of hotels and, working in a straight line, knocked on every door until, around a dozen later, a Mr and Mrs Robbins said yes they would give me a job for the school holidays. I would be a live-in waitress-cum-dogsbody and my pay would be £6 a week, plus tips. Hitching a lift back, I was eager to tell Bessie and Harry what I had done.

They were proud of me. I could tell. I wasn't a soft girl dreaming of education, but someone who was going to go out and work. The only restraint Harry offered was hiring a minibus that August and filling it to the brim with family and friends to visit me.

I told them I was fine, but I wasn't. The snakes had been at my heels again. To keep them off, I'd run daily in the rain along the length of the North Beach. So I was glad to see family and people I knew, and so many of them. Derek, Harry and Bessie themselves, my cousin Olive from 85, and assorted neighbours all smiled like royalty as they stepped carefully on to firm ground to greet me.

When the summer was over, I didn't put the money I'd earned in the bank as I'd planned. Instead, I spent it on a grown-up suit. I bought a dark green tweed, straight-skirted suit, with a square-cut 'boxy' jacket which sat on top of your hips – an Audrey Hepburn suit. To go with it, there was a dark green handbag in mock snakeskin, matching high-heeled shoes and leather gloves. I was sixteen, and looked twenty-five.

What did I do with it? I took it out for walks. About once a fortnight, I put it on, and caught a bus into town. Every now and then I caught two buses to Swansea, where nobody knew me, and studied the twenty-five-year-old version of me reflected in shop windows.

On one of my practising-to-be-a-grown-up outings, I wore the suit to enrol for driving lessons. I couldn't have said then why having a driving licence was so important – but a plan to head off fast into the future needs transport, independence, mobility. I had, in any case, been driving in the African bush since I was thirteen when my friend's father, Old Man Kennedy, had taught me – and I could handle a vehicle well on rough roads, dirt tracks and through herds of wild animals. I only needed to learn traffic and roads.

A few weeks after my seventeenth birthday, I passed my driving test first time out. Puzzled by my skill at such a young age, the examiner asked how I'd learned – quickly regretting it as I launched into the unexpurgated version.

Meanwhile, as that second winter of my A level course gave way to spring and summer, I lagged further behind at school and, ashamed to meet teachers' eyes, bunked off lessons. I took to the countryside, spent hours among trees, walked along river banks and country paths in and out of blackberrying days, guilt and determination, hope and despair pulling me about.

Yes, I would go my own way. I would move and get a job, do anything. I would leave this rural part of Wales, earn money to pay for my freedom and have a new start. Yes, I had broken something when I was a child, or something had been broken for me before I knew how to stop it – something not in my grasp, but still my fault.

The burdens of my past weighing in me, I wanted to start afresh, leave behind my childhood, and I thought you could. I thought you could turn your back on it, like a suitcase crammed full of old stuff left at a bus stop.

But this would mean leaving Harry, and going against his wishes for me. His idea was that an older man would take care of me and children of my own would do the same, bringing me a family, making me belong. But, once married, women stayed at home in Harry's world – a career *or* a husband. How could I explain I wanted both?

I hadn't seen my parents or brother for two years. In East Africa on one of their long contracts, I'd stopped looking forward to the airmail letters they sent. My parents wrote half of the airmail each and sometimes they said nearly the same things. When the letters first started coming, I tore them open, searching for something in them. But there was nothing there. They would write about the weather a bit, about life going on as usual and nothing very much happening. Sometimes they'd report they'd gone to the 'big house' and met the Oppenheimers, who were rich and famous diamond people, or that some important visitors were arriving on the mine.

But my mother didn't draw pictures for me about what she wore, what was happening at the swimming pool, what anyone said, what had made her laugh or what she felt about things. The letters said nothing about my brother either except: 'Chris is well' or 'Chris is well and into everything.' He was six by now, and I couldn't imagine him.

I stopped writing back. My grandmother, who was good at coaxing me, would ask me, gently, to put pen to paper on the odd occasion, which I did, giving as little as I felt I got. As my eighteenth birthday came and went in Wales, I struggled in this limbo of wanting to break free of my past, and not knowing how.

I didn't feel I belonged to anybody any more, and didn't know who had control of me. Did I belong to myself by this time, and did that mean I could step out the door one morning and walk into a grown-up life? Was I in somebody's charge still, or was I free to go?

Then, a chance meeting with a journalist at one of the dances I went to – and I had in my handbag one of my African stories, about Old Man Kennedy. It told of his days as a diamond prospector in Tanzania and our evenings together when he got dressed up for his 'two ladies' and took us to the club house for a drink.

'I've written this,' I said, pushing the pages into the journalist's hand. 'Will you read it and tell me if it's any good?'

A letter a few days later said he thought it was:

'But don't send it to the local press,' he suggested, 'they won't know what to do with it. Aim high.'

I sent my story to Jack Wiggins, editor of the *South Wales Echo* in Cardiff, who seemed high to me.

Ellis the postman was the voice of the village, and an envelope with *South Wales Echo* in bold typeface on the front was too important to trust to the letter box. So he knocked on the door.

'There's a letter for you here, Carol, from the *Echo* in Cardiff.' he said, handing it to me with some solemnity. He then stood his ground while I opened it.

'I've got an interview,' I exclaimed. 'Ooh, I've got an interview for a job – to be a journalist.'

A short while later, our scullery was full. Ellis had knocked on every door in our street where there was post to deliver and told them the news:

'Carol's got an interview for a job on the *Echo* in Cardiff.' People poured into our house and I felt suddenly very important.

Harry fielded the questions, like the ring-master he was, while I stood at the back of the throng watching. It might have been my job interview, but it was his show. 'What's a journalist?' someone wanted to know. Was Cardiff a safe place for a young girl to go by herself? someone else asked.

I rose at 5 a.m. to get ready for the long journey to the capital. The house was peaceful and beguiling at that hour and, waiting for the kettle to boil, I doodled my finger through the salt, sugar and breadcrumbs on the kitchen table, making patterns as I went. Sitting in an armchair a few minutes later with a cup of tea in my hand, I felt at ease in every crease and dust-filled rumple of it.

Not having had an interview before, I didn't know what to expect. It was a chat, it turned out, with Jack Wiggins asking me about myself, about Africa, Egypt, and the fact that my parents and brother were away. Then he asked me when I'd like to start work.

'You're giving me a job!' I exclaimed.

Two weeks on, I had found digs and was working. The editor used my African piece with a picture of me at the top. Travelling back from work on the bus that day, the man next to me had the paper open where I smiled shyly out of it:

'That's me', I said, before I could stop myself. 'I wrote that.'

But already I'd gained an influential enemy. Taking me aside in the corridor when no one else was around, the deputy editor, a man who filled many a reporter with dread, tore my piece to shreds:

'When I become editor I'll make sure you never get another damn thing in the paper,' he said. 'Newspapers are for news, not soppy women's stuff like this.'

God came back during this time – with my father. For a short time in between overseas contracts he came to Cardiff, where my mother had returned to set up house for her, my brother and myself. I welcomed the prospect of another try at family life and was glad to be included in these plans. I wasn't sure, still, what home felt like, missed what I thought it could be: warmth; recognition; – and I wanted to be with my brother.

He had been hit by a Land Rover while overseas and was weeks in hospital having surgery to remove his damaged spleen. None of us knew. My parents hadn't written. But it was the end, for my mother, of being abroad: one child lost to her; the other nearly killed.

Meeting her was a strange, stand-off affair. It had been nearly three years. I was a working woman, taller than her, independent, and anxious to prove it. My brother was different. Chris was seven, and as soon as we saw each other at the railway station in Cardiff, he raced towards me. We hugged excitedly, and I lifted him up and swung him round and round till we were both giddy with laughter.

We liked each other, as we had done before. He held my hand, smiled, and the world felt safe again with my brother by my side. Trust, ease, friendship, softness in his eyes, things I wasn't used to and didn't feel with my parents. He made us a family again.

By the time my father arrived at the end of his contract a few months later, the three of us had made a home and he was the outsider. We had bought second-hand furniture, found workmen, removal men, and got everything in place. I had enjoyed it. I humped furniture around the place, organised my brother to help, smiled at him when my mother got bad-tempered, and enjoyed being calm and in charge. My mother and I were okay too. Never someone I could confide in or talk to, putting the house to rights gave us a practical way of getting on.

I was nineteen when my father came. He rang the front door bell on the afternoon he was expected and I stayed in the back room listening to my mother's matter-of-fact voice asking him what the journey had been like. I had dressed specially. A suit, a cream one bought with my first earnings at the *Echo*, a plain blouse and deliberately high stiletto heels. I was taller than he was when I shook his hand.

It backfired, of course.

'What's this then?' he joked. 'Where's my daughter?'

On another occasion, I was sitting on the arm of my mother's chair, rather large to be doing so, but it was my way of being close to her without knowing how. Staring into the fire, waiting for the door bell to ring to go out with friends, I was wearing what most of us wore at the time – green eyeshadow, masses of backcombed hair and a miniskirt. My father wasn't amused.

'You two will burn in hell,' he suddenly said out of nowhere, glaring at my mother and myself.

Then he went back overseas to start another contract, on his own this time. It was the last time we lived under the same roof. But he left the snakes behind. I thought they'd gone. Now they were here again and by the end of some days, usually in winter, they hissed at my heels and began their writhing in my stomach.

Chris was now eight and the three of us lived in Roath Park near a big open field called the REC, where people played football. It was flat, an ideal place to run, but poorly lit. My mother was worried about me running there alone after work in the dark.

So it was that about once every three or four weeks, when the demons came, I would take my small, friendly brother to help me see off the snakes. We ran, the pair of us, into the darkest spot in the middle of the REC, jumping up and down, waving our arms around, then charging off at full speed towards the path again. We flew along, me chasing him, him chasing me, the snakes, as I discovered years later, chasing us both.

Within two years of the first of these night-time

fleeings, I left Cardiff to work as a reporter on the *Daily Mail* in Manchester, not knowing at the time how much Chris would miss me. I thought only of myself, only of the future. I was leaning on Time again, pushing forwards.

I had the will, as always, to make a fresh start and would spend the next few years rushing, charging on to devour the next event.

'I can do that,' I would say, as I joined my first national newspaper, and I would seldom have a moment to call my own.

Chapter Twenty-Three

‮ঙ‬

THE LAMPLIGHTER

Harry was my nightwatchman for the time I lived in Wales, the ready father of my life, the one who stayed on the ground where I could see him. Waiting for me till I came back from dances or films, he made me cups of tea and chatted before going to bed. But I saw little of him after starting work in Manchester at the age of twenty-one. The journey to West Wales was too long.

Working on the *Mail*, my anxiety, fear of failure, and the feeling of falling apart in my sleep, continued. After visiting the doctor that first time, and getting pills which I threw away, I didn't go back to the surgery.

Then, sometimes, my feeling of loss, of losing myself, happened at the end of the day as well: around evening time. Driving back from a story, along the motorway heading south into Manchester, I'd see people's lighted houses as they slid by. Family scenes: a couple watching

TV; a gathering round a table; a head bent at a kitchen surface; ankles crossed on a sofa; hands held – these images mesmerised me.

They were inside of life, and I was outside, two lots of glass between. Driving in the dark, the light from other people's windows drew me as though I had no lights of my own. In a dream of a moth creature set in a vast prairie, there was miles of blue sky and oceans of long grass, me, the mouse in a cornfield, unworried in my vast surroundings so long as I could see the sun. Then, hawk-like, a giant bird-moth crossed the sun, turning my world dark. The dream returned: me, the mouse running in the long grass; the hawk-like shadow threatening to take my light.

A woman in the office was blind as a bat she said, even with her thick lenses, and I marvelled at the way she walked into a room without seeing more than she had to or being found out. What freedom, I thought, not to be able to focus, not to fear the light going out.

I filled my time with activity: working, going to parties, staying up late, getting up early and working again. I was the all-singing, all-dancing life and soul of many a party. One time a few of us organised a surprise cabaret in a nightclub for a big leaving do. Two reporters going off to jobs in TV, we gave them a good send-off.

Ringing up people on other papers in town, we rounded up the talent. A Sunday paper news editor with a fierce reputation crooned a love song; a night editor on another Sunday did a sketch with his glass eye – lost in the lift on many a drunken night, the orb led an independent life. There was dancing on tabletops, rowdy duets, preposterous jokes, rude impersonations and, as the night wore on, wreaths of fresh flowers came from somewhere and were hung, Hawaiian-style, round our necks.

At a late hour, after pouring myself into a taxi, I got home, undressed – or so I thought – and fell into bed. Hours later I woke carrying with me something of the night before, a bedful of flowers: sweet smelling lilies, freesia, mimosa, carnations – the day's garlands hung on to for once.

The news of my grandfather's death came in a phone call one slow, quiet morning in the office – pneumoconiosis, the miner's disease he'd fought for decades. I sat down with a thump. Harry was the man I called 'Dad' or 'Daddy Williams', the man I didn't want to lose.

I drove straight to Wales where Bessie, my mother, aunts, uncles, cousins were gathered in the scullery of 77. But it was Harry I wanted.

My grandfather's body was upstairs in an open coffin in the back bedroom where he and Bessie had slept. I stood by the big feather bed where as two 'boys' snuggling against him in the dark, Derek and I asked him for more stories.

'Tell us about the War, Dad. What was it like in the War.'

Saturday nights later on, there was Harry stoking the fire to welcome me home in winter. The night he heard my high heels tapping up the street and, when he opened the front door, I slid on the ice and landed, stiff petticoats in the air on the doorstep. The times, in company, he'd proudly put his arm round my shoulders to show me off. The farmers I'd run away from.

I had meant to lean over the coffin, to kiss my grandfather's forehead and hold his hand, but the post-mortem gash starting at his throat was ill-concealed and livid against his thinness, and it threw me back. I sat on the bed where Derek and I had wriggled under the bedclothes like a pair of moles, popping our heads up every now and then for air – and another story.

My grandfather's stories were true, true stories that only happen in the dark, ones where you know your way.

I was twenty-five, the age I had dreamed of being: a flat of my own, a job, a car, but no peace yet, no time to write. None of the calmness of the figure who had urged me on into the future in the mirror of the bedroom next door. The boy's voice then:

'I don't want to be a lady. I want to sleep with you.'

I wasn't allowed to the funeral. In an old Welsh tradition, it was Men Only – as with my grandmother's funeral four years later. While hundreds of dark-coated figures filed through the village up to the chapel, I stayed at home with the women cutting sandwiches and making tea for when people came back to the house.

It was March, and by May I had left the *Mail*. I could not have said why exactly except, raddled by Harry's death, I wasn't able to put a gloss on any more. I wasn't 'happy' and you were supposed to be with what I had. I had an interesting job, my picture in the paper, travel, friends, health, money, prospects, and, by this time, a relationship. Harry would have approved. Gibb was a reporter on the same paper, fifteen years older than me, successful and worldly. No one pushed him around and I liked that. He was his own man.

Falling in love with him within weeks of joining the *Mail*, I enjoyed the fun we had: midnight journeys to Southport for a paddle – and to look for the sea; to Liverpool for fish and chips; to London to stay in the poshest hotel we could find. What I didn't like was the drink. Scotch was *his* demon. Considerate and loving on the one hand, he was maudlin and depressed when I couldn't keep him off it.

I was going away to think, I told him, and no, I didn't know why, except a sense of loss – lowness – and no, he wasn't invited. I was going to the Middle East, to a place called Sharjah, alone.

The choice was to do with how far away and unknown it was – somewhere to lose and find yourself in – and with my mother. A black and white snapshot of her, recalled from my armchair seat, was taken in Sharjah in the United Arab Emirates or the Trucial States as they were then called. Standing strong and straight-backed, shielding her eyes against the desert sun, her expression is one not captured in any other picture. Others have her posed, headachy or giving a wide throwaway smile. Here, she is serene, complete: holding her life.

She had gone there to visit my father on one of his postings to a Forces camp about a dozen miles from Dubai. The picture beguiled me: my mother young and apparently unassailable in her vast, sunlit surroundings; and here I was, about to follow.

Coming across military people who had contacts in Sharjah through the 'killing myself on expenses' series I'd done for the *Mail*, the trip didn't take long to fix. Visa clearance from the local political agent, permission to stay at the Forces base, permission to eat in the Mess were all done quickly.

The editor tried to change my mind. After hedging a bit, I told him some kind of truth: that I was twenty-five years old and felt done in. I'd got everything most people wanted yet I wasn't content. Something was wrong, something I didn't understand, and I wanted to see if I could find out what it was and fix it. If I didn't go now, I never would – and if I came unstuck, well I was young enough to start again.

I didn't tell him the rest, that for the four years I'd worked for him I'd fallen apart in my sleep and maybe there'd be a morning when I'd fail to put myself back together again.

I didn't say either that when I interviewed people, I fell into their stories, and when they stopped, my world went dark. Or that driving back along motorways, I looked for people again in lighted windows in the dark, family scenes along the way.

I was addicted to other people's lives: dangerous stuff.

The risk involved in the location I was flying to didn't hit me till the presence, at my farewell party, of people I realised, suddenly, I didn't want to leave: Thompson, a special friend, Shelley, Mike, Pete, Malcolm, Pat, Celia, – and Gibb himself. With his farewell gift of a hipflask – to be carried at all times, in case I got lost in the desert – Thompson took me aside, held me, told me not to stay away too long, and to be sure to come back.

I was leaving all this friendship, care, love to go somewhere hot, dry, inhospitable and politically sensitive; to a country reputedly unfriendly to women where I didn't speak the language, where there were few Europeans, and where I would be living alone.

If I rang tomorrow I could have my job back. For a moment it seemed the thing to do, but it was too late. I'd severed the tie which had held me and the office together in four unbroken years.

Chapter Twenty-Four

❧

THE BLUE LAMP

Renzo is moving his family from France to Clapham, on the south side of London, from where he can get to Maidstone fairly quickly.

In the house in Clapham, it falls to his wife, whose English is not yet good, to deal with workmen. A saga develops over the bathroom and heating. I offer a reliable plumber and central heating firm.

Sharjah was hot – 120° in the shade. I arrived at night to a blanket of warmth and a heady mix of the smell of sand, heat, sea. Getting the taxi to drive along the waterfront, I looked at the lights and stopped to hear the sound of waves lapping on the quayside. It was going to be all right, I thought. The smell of the air, and its warmth dampening my skin, cloaking my hair, drew me in, included me.

I was the sole occupant of the old disused fort on the

edge of the camp at Sharjah where only a few years previously two Egyptian men, with special dispensation from Cairo, had been flogged over the black cannons for raping a local woman. The fort stood three-quarters of a mile away from the camp. So no traffic came, no jeeps or trucks, no lights, no trees, no human voices.

My first three nights were hell. Surrounded by sand, I sat in my room at night buried, the silence of sand and the heavy air like a tomb. Peace and quiet is what I'd wanted. This felt like death and my mind set up a clamour against it, like an insurrection.

Why had I done this to myself? Nobody had forced me. Why had I removed all the safe, comfortable props in my life to plant myself here, on the tip of a vast Saudi-Arabian land mass? Why had I left a bustling city, a busy job, friends, newspapers, phone, TV, radio, buses, taxis? And now that I'd buried myself among billions and trillions of grains of sand, could I get out again and still save face? Could I leave and say I'd made a mistake?

No, I couldn't. I had to see it out.

I learned over the next few months that a desert has different kinds of silences and if you don't yield to them, they can drive you mad. In those first three nights, a gale of protest in my head rose against the wall of soundlessness. Never had I known such commotion in my mind. There was clattering, screeches to set your teeth on edge, percussion din and the fear I would never know relative peace, order or quiet again.

In the fort I had two sparsely furnished connecting rooms: a bedroom and a living room, both with old stone walls. On my second night, I was trying to read and, on impulse, got up and stood facing the wall, my fingertips pressed lightly against the rough surface; toes too. I wanted to climb. I wanted to be on the ceiling, away from all this, not down here. Up there, I wouldn't feel this way. I'd escape.

Shocked to be thinking such thoughts, I stood there a long while, still and quiet, my nose millimetres from the wall's surface. I knew I wanted to climb the wall and knew I mustn't try. Staying there on the edge until I grew tired, then walking away, several more times that evening the wall drew me back. Only near it was my mind quiet. I had equilibrium here, a sense of poise even.

Facing the wall on the third night; the balance was delicate but clear, a fine line between stillness – paying attention – and madness – climbing. Felt in the lightness of the pressure of fingertips against stone, it lay in distance too, in how far my face was from the wall's surface and in the exact positioning of my feet. Keeping them all in balance, I was safe, calm. Urges to pound the wall, to slump against it, to cry or to pace the floor had to be resisted. My usual ways of escape – making a song and dance, flying, climbing, floating or fighting – wouldn't do.

We didn't talk about grief in our family and, in a dream,

objects lost from my childhood float on a calm sea. Sleeping in the fort at Sharjah, my night eyes know the shipwreck has already happened and the storm is over. Now the jetsam from it lies, bobbing around gently on smooth water — miniature furniture from the doll's house, toys, paint boxes, crayons, a blackboard and easel, animals. It isn't only Harry's death, it's years of loss.

On the fourth night of sitting alone with my books and notebooks, my impulse to climb the living-room wall has gone and I'm peaceful. I haven't climbed out of my body to float on the ceiling: it's grief, and I have to stay home for it.

I begin to hear small normal noises in the night, rustlings of creatures and insects. Even in a fort in a desert surrounded by sand, there are shiftings, stirrings, movement and noise. The sound of the ceiling fan in the bedroom is like the one in Egypt: whirring; pushing air through its large blades.

The English-speaking community at Sharjah was small enough for people to have heard I was coming. They'd thought I was suffering jet lag, so my emergence on my fourth or fifth day was about right. Eating at the mess and being introduced to people in the civilian community, soon I found companions for walks, swimming, fishing and exploring. One, a meteorologist called Bryan, appointed himself my guide, making sure I was taken around safely and listening to me talk about the man I had left behind. An easy companion, he swam like a dolphin, bringing fish and coral back from the reef.

Once we got lost in the desert and asked directions at a sheik's summer palace where, spending the day, I was invited to swim alone in a beautiful mosaic pool. Shaded from the hot sun by an arbour of vine leaves, perfumed blossom and exotic climbing plants, it was watered from an underground spring.

Lying on my back floating, the sun glinted through leaves and petals and, at my side, large fish swam. A giant aquarium inside the palace ran the whole length of the pool, separated only by thick glass, so it seemed you swam with the fish alongside you, some the size of small sharks.

Over the weeks I watched the desert from various vantage points and saw it turn through seven shades one evening, each distinct, before slipping into night. Soon I felt safe to walk alone along the shoreline where there were dozens of miles of deserted beach.

Life settled into a rhythm. Early morning being the only cool time, I was up with the sun and drinking coffee on the fort ramparts within minutes of my eyes opening. Lunchtimes and evenings were spent with other people, Bryan often picking me up and escorting me to the mess or out to dinner. Mornings and afternoons I spent alone, my 'thinking' time.

A few times a week, getting an early lift to the nearby beach in an army truck, I'd walk and enjoy the morning before it got too hot. For protection, I'd bought long loose, Arab-style clothing in the local souk. The sea breeze billowed these soft cottons around me and kept me cool. I enjoyed the floating sensation and sometimes this and the empty beach made me feel like a dhow on the shoreline.

What I now think of as 'the day the lamp arrived' began ordinarily enough with an early morning walk along the shore: white sand; blue sea; blue sky; and the breeze making sails out of my billowing clothes. I stopped to look at a small insect burrowing in the sand and felt myself falling. Not frightening, but distinct. Still standing upright where I was, I was falling, down, down into a deep place, through the sand, through the bottom of the earth, wherever that is, and out through the sky at the other side. It took perhaps a few seconds. I didn't tell anyone about it and went, as usual after these walks, to the beachside house of a British diplomat to lunch with his wife who then, as usual, drove me back to the fort.

By that evening of my journey through the centre of the earth I was carrying a lamp inside my stomach – also distinct. An ornate affair, shiny gold, with a long spout, it was from a child's storybook, an Aladdin's cave type of lamp a genie would spring from. But instead of a genie, a blue flame.

I accepted it without question, this lamp in my stomach, and it would take me years to understand what it was, what it meant: that I had conjured it, like an intuitive gift, to see me through my grieving. I wanted back my magic grandfather with his true stories and words to make our night eyes shine. I wasn't ready to let him go.

At the time the lamp was as real to me as the sentences I wrote in my reporter's notebook, the cannons on the ramparts, or the sun coming up. It had a blue flame which burned evenly and constantly, day and night, for almost exactly a year. In that time, it never left my stomach, flickered or moved in any way. Whatever I might be doing – working, shopping, swimming, staring quietly at the ceiling – it was there.

My claim to something I could keep through the night, it remained with me from one day through to the next, constant and trustworthy like the nightwatchman I had lost. Steadily lit, I began to like waking at night, to enjoy being still and peaceful in the dark. And by day, I was calm, serene even, with the lamp to guide me.

The day the lamp left me, tough decisions were hardening in my mind. Living back in Manchester for almost a year, the offer of a TV contract came in a phone call one afternoon – in a place I had never wanted to live: London. Frightening and anonymous as the Big City seemed, I had to consider the prospect. The move would fit in with other decisions: to leave full-time journalism and take a step towards writing books.

But quitting Manchester? All my friends, and the city itself – so much of me scattered in fragments around it. There was scarcely a corner of it I hadn't found or written a story on. I'd worked it hard.

It was harder by far to leave Gibb. Part of me loving him still, how could I go? But neither my absence in the Middle East nor my presence in the last year had made things right between us.

On the day the lamp left, I woke early and looked at the higgledy-piggledy suitcases on top of the wardrobe. I knew this was it: I would pack them today – and go to London. At that moment, just after dawn, the lamp went out. The inside of my body was dark again and I knew I had to manage on my own.

Moving to London, I eventually buy the house where I watch home videos years later from my armchair and see the lamp again for the first time since that Manchester morning. It's in a North London terrace of three-storey houses with two and a half rooms on each floor.

Shortly after buying it, a new friend called Sally moves in for a while and we split the space. I take the bottom of the house, she the top, and we share a bathroom and kitchen in between. In her mid-twenties with blonde hair and large blue eyes, Sally is wise beyond her years and fun to be with. Serious or laughing, sharing with her is easy.

Work is not. When my year's TV contract ends, instead of renewing it, I come home to write my first book, but it won't shape up. I've written hundreds of articles, and hundreds of thousands of words, but the book defeats me. As do London tubes. Claustrophobia is pressing in and I can't any more pretend it isn't.

I'm split in two inner rooms again – sunshine and darkness – living in the house where, a decade later, I will rent space from the new owner, Sue. The Sunshine Room inside me is discovering London; making new friends; sharing with Sally; films; theatre; trips to the sea.

Darkness is the book, the London Underground, long hours spent at the desk trying to work, trying to find my way. It's the return of the feeling I fall apart each night and start the day from scratch. I decide to seek help.

A colleague suggests a woman psycho-analyst who lives not far from me. We speak. It's July, the analyst is going off on holiday, and we agree to start work in September.

Waking up early on a morning in August, eighteen months after Sally had moved in, I knew something was badly wrong. Not something fallen apart inside me, but not far off, something in the house. A Sunday, I knew Sally was at her boyfriend's about a mile away – or perhaps she'd come back again? Someone was moving stealthily around. I looked at the clock: 5.30 a.m. Sally slept in the room above mine and I went there first. It was empty – and the rest of the house too, secure and still. I went back to bed.

Half an hour later I woke to a huge crashing of glass, as though all the windows in the house had shattered and fallen to the floor. The clock showed 6 a.m. The crash seemed to have started above me. Heart thudding, I raced upstairs to Sally's room again. Untidy as always, it was still quiet, empty – and the windows intact. All round the house there was not a crack in a window pane, nothing amiss.

But something was. Getting dressed, I went round the house again, out into the garden to peer up at the roof and onto the street at the front to look at the houses next door. I was back inside drinking coffee when the door bell rang. Richard, Sally's boyfriend, was standing there, bent over, keening softly like a wounded animal. Sally was dead.

She had woken at 5.30, as I had, with an unexpected cough. When it wouldn't stop, she had gone outside for air. It was hot and humid that summer and Richard thought nothing of it, but she came back in a short while insisting he call an ambulance. 'I can't breathe,' she said.

In the time it took him to realise how serious she was, and to get to the phone, she was pacing the floor. As 999 kept ringing with no answer, she got more agitated, and he tried to calm her. Cursing the delay, he kept on looking at the clock. At 6 a.m., when I'd woken to the sound of breaking windows in the house, she crashed over his large glass coffee table, shattering it in pieces. She was dead before the ambulance arrived.

Sally was twenty-seven, and a post-mortem showed she died from her first attack of asthma. None of us, least of all Sally herself, knew she had it. An only child, her mother had died the Christmas before. Sally's father had to be told straight away. He lived in South Africa and would take some time to arrive. They had been very close, laughter from upstairs letting me know when he was on the phone to her.

He stayed a fortnight, long enough to hear the daily stories of the last eighteen months of Sally's life. He wanted to know as many of them as I could relate and in as much detail as I could remember. We sat at restaurant tables late into the night and laughed a lot. I could see why Sally liked him so much. He was kind, funny, dignified – and a marvellous listener. He met her friends, spent time with Richard and, finally, when he felt the picture of Sally's life up to the morning she died was whole, he said it was time to leave.

I missed him. Warmed by his kindness and care, I made comparisons, too, between his relationship with Sally and the way I had grown up.

It wasn't until he'd gone I discovered how guilty I felt to be alive while Sally was dead. She was a few years younger than me, funnier, more carefree – and loved for all of her life by her father. How – why – should I, without love like that, be alive when she was gone?

The fear of my dark room returned in force. Sally had vanished, disappeared on me. She'd gone where I couldn't see or find her and my empty house was like a morgue.

Throwing myself into work, walking a lot, in and out of rooms, up and down stairs, I hoped to tire myself enough to sleep. Waking at night, I did the same, standing in Sally's room in the dark sometimes, I gazed at the garden. She used to lie in it on hot weekends, and while Sally lay outside, I sat inside at my desk in the cool and shade of the basement. There were open French windows between us leading from the back of the basement room out into the small garden and I wandered out every now and then to sit with her.

My brother, now at university, is shocked by Sally's death, as are my parents. Settled in Cardiff in the house they bought when I worked on the *Echo*, my mother especially is shaken. Staying with me from time to time, remarking more than once on Sally's untidiness; I can tell how much she now regrets it.

About a month after Sally's death, shortly after her father had gone, I was at my desk. It was another warm day, but with summer drawing to an end and the French windows closed. Behind with work, broke and despairing, I had no heart for the garden, or for anything. Struggling, I set to writing an article for a Sunday paper: long, complicated and overdue. Looking up some time later, it was sunny – and there was Sally standing in her white bathing suit outside the French windows, smiling. Then she was gone.

I reached for the phone to dial a friend's number. 'What happens to people when they die?' I asked Peter. 'Where do they go? They can't just disappear.'

People didn't, he said to me. They were held in trust by the rest of us. When I'd grieved, she would remain: me, and others, as her witness. But I wasn't any good at grieving, I told him. That was my life. No good at holding on to things I'd lost. I didn't keep them. They went away from me.

And it was Sally's *physical* presence I missed, it was swimming with her, cooking, drinking a glass of wine, and being teased for my seriousness. That's what I wanted, not a memory. I missed her voice, her laugh, her calmness. I missed everything about her that was gone.

Urging me to get away he said it was an insult – to myself – to be sitting trying to work.

In an Indian summer that year, the sun hurt my eyes with its shining. Walking on a Welsh beach, I wanted winter to come fast, to be able to hide. Sally had gone into the dark where I couldn't find her and I never wanted the sun to shine again.

By the end of that late summer and its dazzling days, I had walked Welsh hills and beaches long enough and hard enough for something to move inside me. A thin shaft of light had pushed through into the cave I was holed up in.

Using that light over the following months, and the torch which therapy provided, I explored the dark place inside myself and the coils, loops and luggage stored in it from long ago. It wasn't easy. Sometimes my bleakness drove me back with excuses like: I had no right to be alive with Sally gone, why bother? Other times, I was afraid to venture, alarmed by what I felt or saw. My fear of the snakes' hissing and the piled-up boxes drove me back again to the surface where things were smooth and safe.

Running out into the tennis courts, the park, the fresh air, work, anywhere away from the darkness, I held off. But, things were turning inwards. It was autumn, getting cold, and there was no more sun in the garden.

Chapter Twenty-Five

~જી

MURDER IN THE FAMILY

Renzo is cheerful. He says my body is responding to our combined efforts to help it. My sternum is yielding at last and my breathing improved. He's jaunty almost.

I'm not. I want my life back, the one where I was able-bodied – and useful. Pain lessened now to twinges and small aches, how much more time and trust will it take before I can work again? It's been more than a year and I am still not myself: no spontaneous movements; limited use of my hands; slow walking; the feeling, still, that a jolt or nudge would dislodge me.

At the cinema show in my armchair, the next vivid picture is of a dark-haired girl – but she's not me.

On a summer's day in the year following Sally's death I'd gone to fetch a paper and was walking back to the house when a neighbour's child, Caroline, raced up to say hello. She was three, a pretty, gregarious child with shiny hair and big brown eyes. We were good pals, and I picked her up to take her inside. Walking down the steps to the basement door, we moved from sunshine into shade and, all of a sudden, something fell across me, a shadow, like a blanket, thrown from behind. Quickly, I raced back up the steps and took Caroline home.

Once inside my own house, I began to 'erupt' like a volcano, as if my body would break into thousands of small pieces. It went on for about an hour. When it subsided, I sat at last. I knew what it was. It had been heading my way since I'd begun therapy the previous autumn, like a hurricane I'd been trying to dodge.

'Why are you so afraid of anger?' I'd been asked.

'I'm *not*,' I insisted, and went on denying it, claiming I wasn't the sort of person who stored up anger from the past. But I was.

The shadow on the steps of my house was my father as he had seemed to me as a child, his sudden appearances behind me causing my world to fall apart: rooms jumping up at me; settees growing out of size; my father as high as the church where he and his God made the rules. His voice was like a death knell and at its first strike, the mother of the dolls used to 'die'.
So I was angry.

A short time before the 'volcano', I'd told the analyst about my father being a blight on my playtimes, about the spilled milk and the jokes that went wrong in Ncema Dam. I'd also told her about losing myself at night, how

I was waylaid by bad dreams like falling among thieves, how they stole my confidence. Each morning I had to pick up the pieces, put myself back together again, find what I was for and why. But what I left out was that this happened *every time* I went to sleep, not just occasionally. I woke undone, unravelled every day.

If I would 'listen' to the dreams, she said, and learn what they were telling me, they would lose their alarming power. They were trying to get me to take notice, that's all.

But I was afraid the humiliating, menacing, terrifying bits of my past would overwhelm me if I acknowledged them. How could I stop them doing that? How, in the present, do you treat with thieves from the past who have the power to undo you?

The nightmare was this:

I was in a concrete coffin, but breathing – buried alive – my punishment for being bad. Pinned on my back, unable to move, I was to stay like this for ever, never to leave the coffin, nor to die. A male figure tended this death-life, feeding me oxygen through a single straw. I didn't see his face, but my breathing depended on him.

This is what I feared not coming back from, why I couldn't believe in myself till my arms, legs, head were moving proof of my freedom from its paralysing grip. Unremembered at the time, the figure in this coffin nightmare had been with me in Wales when, as a sixteen-year-old living with Harry and Bessie, a shadowy hunched shape had charge of my oxygen supply.

Waiting to catch me out as soon as I lost consciousness, these night-time torments threatened my life, terror of them undermining me. Keeping myself short of sleep to see if I could avoid them, I went to bed late and got up early.

'Why do you have to get up at six every morning?' a friend asked. Unspoken answer: to try and stop my dreams.

The nightmare of being buried alive in this way began a few years before Sally died. It let me know my time was up. An inner life of inhabiting different rooms, memories kept in boxes, terror underneath, claustrophobia, writers' block, had to be confronted. I could not hide from myself any longer.

At some time during my first few weeks of therapy I talked of the block which stopped me producing my first book, not yet seeing the link with claustrophobia: my fear of being trapped in a lift while the words were trapped in me. The analyst had said:

'You know, you are stopping yourself from writing because you are afraid it would be like murdering your father.'

'What!' This was double Dutch to me and seemed to confirm the rumour you hear about these people – they're batty themselves. Murdering my father – what nonsense.

But it's true – and takes years to accept – the violence

and murder in our smooth-on-the-surface family. For I have two fathers, one in the house, and one in the Old Testament. She's missed out an 'S', that's all. And, yes, I want my second father dead for what he's done to me. He's alibied my father in the crime of trying to make me perfect – a girl for God. So, yes, patricide was on my mind. Murder in a family is catching.

Getting older, fighting for my life and sanity, I tried to kill this God many times. I had to. He was heartless – and I needed love in order to survive. Inhuman, making of me a woman barely breathing in a coffin, there was no love in Him, only a demand for perfection – and I wanted a life. I had to win.

Yet, hopelessness lay at the heart of all my rows over religion with my real father: guilt at how dreadfully wrong they were; despair that I could not seem to stop them or make things right. With God on his side, there was always a punishment, a threat, my father could get me with, a shark circling in the water:

'You'll be sorry, my girl. Just you wait and see.' Simple words, but they never failed to bring me down, speaking as they did of the other Father in the wings. They pulled me under for twenty years or more, for whenever love, peace of mind, success beckoned, I didn't believe they were mine to grasp.

Therapy had ended and incapacity began before I was ready to see my father and his God as what they were – the same person, his God my father's invention. Before then, it was a fight to the death between my father and me, our conflicting stories, our versions of the truth, like a tug-o-words between us: the Old Testament at one end and a child's story at the other. Or, so I thought.

But no. There were two children on the rope.

My father's God was given to him when he was around four or five years old and staying in the orphanage, where he was put when his mother was ill. His two sisters, being older than him, were allowed to stay at home with their father, Owen. But Owen was frail and unable to manage the needs of a young child. So my father was sent into care.

Recalling what a miserable place the local orphanage was, my aunt said: 'Once you handed a child over, that was it. You gave up any rights. You could visit once a week and that's all you were allowed.' The thinking was that contact with parents would upset a child – which is just what happened one day.

The children were taken once a week to church, marching silently there in a crocodile. On one of these Sunday outings, my father spotted Owen on the other side of the road where he was standing, semi-hidden, hoping for a glimpse of his son.

'Dad', he shouted, breaking ranks. 'Dad.'

Caught when he was halfway across the road, he was boxed about the ears, shoved back into line and marched away.

This image of his son, hit about the head and marched on, haunted Owen. Speaking of it to my aunt, he said he would always remember his son's cries, and the anguish of letting him down.

After this, Owen was told it was best for him not to visit my father at all because it upset the boy so much. The person who visited instead was a family friend called Walter. My aunt recalls Walter as a nice man, but remembers, too, his preoccupation with a fire-and-brimstone Creator. This was the God Walter gave his young charge in the orphanage. A blood-curdling account of a God of testing vengeance was thought to be what was needed to make my father strong and able to withstand his bleak times.

When he returned home, my father seemed normal: happy to be back in the family; playing football; getting up to mischief; annoying his sisters.

As with Nellie's childhood, I learn the story of my father's God by my aunt's hearth in Maidstone. She brings me old photographs: of my father as a boy; of the three of them together, him and his sisters; of their mother as a young woman; their father in a bowler hat. My mind is full.

In the couple of years following Sally's death I start to write seriously: a piece about her to begin with. Printed in the *Sunday Times*, hundreds of readers respond to it.

What with grief, work and therapy, I remove myself from my family for a while, declare myself an orphan. When occasional visits to Wales resume, I've changed more than I realise and it's noticed. Coming to understand that religion is my father's life, his reason to be alive, I know I can't, mustn't, take this away from him. I mustn't demolish his God. So I don't.

Refusing to engage as I did in the past, if my father criticises and shouts, I say nothing and move away. I won't fight. If things start up, I stand aside. It's not my war. There is a difference, too, in my bearing, my step, something subtle and too obvious to ignore. The lens in my mind's eye has turned somehow. On one occasion, listening to him rage, he seems to grow distant from me, becoming smaller, as he had once, when I was a child, become bigger.

For a while, with me 'gone' like this, and come home to myself at last, my father's God seems to trouble him more. He sits, head in hand, Bible open, trying to read, but he can't. The words won't link together. He knows what they are as they stand on their own, but they refuse to form sentences, and however long he looks at the page, he can't make them.

He rings me to ask for help. He wants a reading list of books I think he might get on with. But where to begin with a man who's only known one testament? He's had nothing to read in the house for a long time, no newspapers, no magazines, a copy of the Bible, that's all, and the romantic fiction my mother skims. Books *I've* written, which I used to send, were either given away or lost – 'too difficult' for them to read. So I stopped sending.

Now, I try my best. A reading list is sent through the post. I hear nothing back – and do not ask.

The small miracle, when it happens, is barely noticed. My father who for more than thirty years has been deaf to my words, is moved by my silence. He wants my opinion one day. It's the first time.

'Do you believe in hell?' he phones to ask me.

'No,' I reply, and say no more. I understand at last what I'm struggling with: my hell is my business and my father's is his.

Chapter Twenty-Six

❧

TUG-O-WORDS

Therapy was a long business and I was defensive, afraid to unpick the gnarled knots in my life's story. I wouldn't deconstruct myself for fear of not having an identity if I did. Hell was so strong in me, I held on to it as what I knew, wanting rid of it on the one hand – and frightened to let go of its security on the other.

Then there was my impatience. I wanted to get on with things, move forwards, see results. Once something was spotted – like anger – I thought it was grasped and wouldn't wait for it to settle. I had forgotten too much of Africa, of my patience as a child in the bush waiting for a flick of a dik-dik's tail or a glimpse of its wet muzzle.

I wanted – needed – to believe in myself as an adult, for I had a life to lead. I wrote for national newspapers, owned a house, appeared on TV, lectured in public, gave seminars at universities. But with the analyst I was a terrified child who didn't want to pay attention and wouldn't meet her gaze. Treating her like I'd treated Nellie, I kept my distance and ran away. Dashing back in time, I picked up whatever was to hand, threw episodes from the past at her, often out of sequence, then retreated.

One day, she caught me, though, held me before I could run again, for there was something else I'd had to defend myself against besides giants. Where was my mother when it was going on: the partings; my father's punishments; God; Nellie? Where was she? Why didn't she save me? Did she comfort me at all? Did I tell her things, confide in her?

I blocked the questions to begin with. How did I know where my mother was? Sometimes she was ill with nerves and migraines. Sometimes she was busy. Sometimes she didn't know what was going on. But the walls around me were beginning to crumble. My adult self not up to the task of seeing what lay behind them, it was a child's voice which began my mother's story – in Ncema Dam, the lost paradise we lived in when I was nine.

'I did that. I muzzled a growling dog, snapped its mouth shut till its teeth rattled.'

'And when did you do that?' the analyst asked.

'When I was an African child.'

'So tell me about Africa.'

'I used to steal things. I stole piano lessons in Africa because I wanted to learn to play and I forged my father's signature to get lessons in boarding school.

'I stole things when I was a Welsh child too. I stole butter from my Nana's pantry for our dens in the woods, and potatoes from Harry's sack and Harry and Bessie were poor . . .'

'I'm frightened of the box,' the English child said and, then:

'My mother didn't rescue me – and she never said "sorry".'

With God and my father at least I could be angry. What to do, though, about a mother I loved?

But then, my mother's fairy-tale version of my childhood had distressed me for years. Talking to her as an adult about my young life, she denied any – all – of the darkness in it. I was never locked in a trunk. That was my brother and he'd laughed about it. I had never been ill, or had cerebral malaria or been sent away for years. And the changes of schools? Surely there weren't that many.

My mother had denied my experiences when I was a child too. As I tried to put the jigsaw together, to make pictures out of the jumbled pieces of my life, my mother told me what I saw and what had happened to me wasn't true. If I talked about events in the places we'd been, she told me I'd imagined them:

There was no shooting in the streets in Suez.
Mr van J was a nice man.
Nana Lee was kind to me.
I didn't carry a gun.

Yet still I needed to protect my mother. There had to be one safe place in my past. I wasn't ready. I'd learned to live without a father's love, but betrayal by my mother? No.

The therapist was persistent. I had arrived at her doorstep on my knees almost, a combination of writers' block and claustrophobia making my life unworkable: and out on my knees she sent me many a time, to think again. And again.

She said, one day, as I continued to play my desultory game of hide and seek with the past: 'A mother's love, or its inadequacy can give or take away from us the possibility of "living" in its fullest sense. This is the loss you are afraid of. You can see off – so to speak – the giants of God and your father, yet you are still afraid to face how your mother has let you down.'

It still seems too much for me to bear. Then a dream:

I am waiting in a house to be taken away to be executed. I can't remember the crime I've committed, but I know, in dread, I can't undo it. I can't go back and change the past, and now I face death because of it.

But, then I am reprieved. The *female* executioner doesn't come to take me away and as time passes I know I am free to leave. I go to a florist's and there a woman companion buys a daffodil as a buttonhole – the flower of Wales, where my mother and I were born.

But there's still something from the 'Eden' of Ncema Dam which is disturbing me. It's something to do with snakes. They chased me till I left 'home' for good at the age of twenty-one. I didn't hear one after that. What was it with these snakes?

It was Harry, to begin with. One night, after my ninth birthday and shortly before my first visit to Africa, he had a story for Derek and me:

'There was once a man who went to Africa. He was travelling through the jungle, and decided to have a little rest. So he sat down on a tree trunk – and guess what?'

We couldn't of course.

'The next thing he knew, the tree trunk started to move, and it was a big, big snake he was sitting on, so big it was as high as the biggest tree you've ever seen, and it turned round and swallowed him up. And do you know what? It even swallowed his handkerchief. Now, there's a hungry snake for you.'

'Will there be lots of snakes in Africa?' I asked Harry, before going out the door of 77 that night to sleep at 85.

'Hundreds,' he said. 'Thousands. Some of them big as trees.'

Sleeping at my cousin's, my nightmare of being chased by hundreds of snakes who were going to eat me alive woke me up. There was only one thing to do – run for it. I was halfway down the street in my plaid dressing gown when a woman took hold of my hand.

'Where are you going, bach?' she asked.

'I'm running away,' I said. 'I don't want to go to Africa because I'm frightened of all the snakes.'

'And where do you live?'

'I live at number 77 – but I'm sleeping at 85.'

I liked snakes when we lived in Africa, liked watching them sliding S-shaped along the lawn. They made my mother shriek and I felt grown-up, her being silly and me not being afraid of them.

So why was I taking so long?

I see a picture of a snake in our bathroom at Ncema Dam, a spitting cobra. The middle of the night, I'd been woken by commotion in the house and was standing in pyjamas at the bathroom door. The snake was in the bath, coiled round in a loop at the bottom, its head rearing. My father raised a heavy, gnarled stick and with one blow killed it. Hanging on to a surface in the kitchen, head down, swaying, my mother was silent as my father shouted:

'They're evil – and it's her – ' pointing at me – 'she invites them in with those lizards of hers. She'll be the death of us.'

For the first time I speak of the curse which I didn't know I suffered from, which followed me from the coffin nightmare into my waking hours: if I ever told anyone about the nightmare, then it would come true. I would be 'taken' – and buried alive for ever, snatched away from life and never rescued.

This was the snake I couldn't see, which slid between wake and sleep, night and day: my father's wrath on the one hand; my mother's frailty on the other; me the bad child bringing death – a snake in the bath to prove it.

Years of furled-up terror are spoken at last, fears I wasn't aware of: that badness and failure were in me, like the hiss of a serpent. Doom was in my body. I couldn't escape it – and no one could save me. Guilt, too, pours out. I think the poison is unstoppable, me the woman-snake of my father's prophecy, the family's despair and unhappiness my fault.

The hold with which my father tried to keep me silenced – and weakened – was: Thou Shalt Not Tell. Sworn to silence like this, the coffin lay 'real' and intangible inside me. For years it kept me subdued and away from my strength and vital life. I could not, would not, admit what I knew – that I was guilty, bad, terrified – and hostage to a box.

Trying to piece my life together as an adult, eighteen changes of school, partings, endings, gaps, being lost have done for my sense of narrative. My parent's on-off marriage, the struggle with finding and losing things over the years, I feel like an incident zone, invisible between one event and the next, no thread to connect me.

What I had wanted back from the villains of my childhood was my memory – the story of my life. Yet, I had also avoided knowing it, protecting myself from the pain. So there is still the history of my life to fit together, to give me the sense of continuity I long for – and am also afraid of. The child's voice from a long time back comes through: a god-defying, determined, pencil-hoarding girl.

There was evidence, from when I was four, that I wouldn't go quietly. Language, words, pictures, stories – added up day by day, they grew in my den. Done in though I was on the one hand, I'd pop back for another go on the other.

A Jill-in-a-box kind of child, flattened one minute, singing and dancing the next, I'd shown signs of being someone who would say her piece. Put down, sworn to silence, smacked, shut in a trunk, I would not keep my mouth shut for long. Yes, I had defiance in mind – and also memory. It was kept.

The person who built the walls and kept the pencils and the rhythms in her head safe was a child who had started defending the details of a life from the age of three or four, and she hadn't let up.

Behind the deep wall of the den which my childhood self has built, dynamite sticks of anger lie side by side with strands of memory. Ammunition and pencil stubs lie criss-crossed and I can't get at one without the other.

My story is wrapped in a time bomb, rage for the neglect, the waste, of my childhood in the same spot as the memory of it. If I learn it, it might kill me, I am that angry.

Writers' block. A story that can't find its way through the wall.

Despair begins to ease at last and there's space inside me. Dreaming of the actual physical house where I live, I begin to move up the stairs, away from the basement into an attic room where there's air and sunlight. I also have the first night-time flight where I soar over the countryside like a human glider. There are dreams of vividly coloured birds and exotic animals. One night there's a creature which is a cross between an elephant, a rhinoceros and an African fish eagle.

There's difficulty too, a dream where I know where the light switch is, but can't turn it on. It's *my* hand, though. It's not blame on the outside that's needed to save a life, but work – and light – on the inside.

Talking to my brother I find he, as an adult, has snakes, demons and troubles of his own: a difficult career – in my father's footsteps – and a feeling of not knowing his way.

'Change now if you want,' I urge him. 'If you do it now, you'll have time. You can stay with me. We'll manage.'

But engineering is something Chris is good at and it's what he knows.

By the time therapy ends, I have begun to acknowledge what the resourceful, affectionate child of my young self has kept for me behind her defences. She's not a murderer in fact. Neither is she someone to be thwarted in the long-term by giants – not even one as big as me.

'If this is the shape of the world I have come into,' this child had said at one point, 'then I shall have a jungle of my own, a garden which nobody else can see.'

Looking for what she has done years later, I find that behind the high walls, in another one of her secret places, she has grown beds of huge, scarlet poppies. Masses of red, the colour of life-saving blood and anger.

These are the main flowers in the back garden of the house I am living in. They were there when I arrived, and I liked their boldness so much I took seeds from the dead heads of them that first year, dug them in and scattered them around. Sally had laughed at me for making so much work of it.

'They'll be like triffids,' she'd said.

Now, in the summers following her death, they are huge, wild and all over the garden.

Chapter Twenty-Seven

❧

THE CENTIPEDE STORY

I do not whisper a word of my childhood stories to Renzo who, fifteen months into the incapacity, works on my body. I have told him I've been through therapy and warned him off dabbling in my emotions. But we have been together for eight months and my desire to kick him in the shins has gone. Instead, as he treats me, I ask him questions about bodies and about osteopathy. I had no idea, for example, that the body has upwards of 600 muscles which have the job of keeping bones and sockets in place, as well as providing muscle power of their own.

I had no idea, either, that when muscles *do* 'muscle in' during an injury, they subtly change shape. Their leaning over a bit to take on extra work costs them. My own compounded injury was caused by years and years of muscles and the tissues connecting them being put under stress and bent out of shape from trying to keep my body – me – going. And for all of my life, bones are what I thought I had. As long as none of *those* were broken, I carried on regardless.

It's obvious from our long conversations that Renzo's view of the body is different from most people's. To him it is a balanced and intelligent organism, something to be worked with and learned from, which carries within itself the means of its own health and repair.

'We feel things in the body,' he said one day. 'That is why we should listen. That is how we learn.'

'I've become fond of muscles,' I say. 'I think they're brave and obliging, but why is the link between them and emotions so vital?'

He takes a deep breath:

'When we are hurt somewhere in the body we can choose not to feel the pain or, if it's emotional, we can forget the event which caused it. In this way, we can forget a small part of our body, a muscle, perhaps a series of small muscles and fascia. So, this part of the body is in your body, but not fully integrated, because you have forgotten about it.'

With what he calls 'complex injuries', Renzo's job, he says, is to reintegrate the forgotten part into the mind. Then, as he sees it, the mind and body work together to bring about the necessary healing which the mind by itself has chosen to turn its back on. The mind, he says, often refuses to remember, and the body reminds it. He gives an example of a woman who had a pain in her hip, which meant she could not move one of her legs outwards.

'I did a normal treatment with no result at all. And one day she said: "I remember when I was a little girl, I was hurt by the fence. I was trying to climb on it, and I got stuck, and it hurt my hip. It's funny because I never remembered this until the last session when you were working on my hip." And from this moment, she could open the hip. She could not open that leg before because she was protecting the area which was hurt.'

I ask, in that case, what osteopathy does physically that other treatments don't.

'We have to give the body the chance to be its own doctor,' he says. His purpose is to bring back the normal range and quality of movement the body had before it was injured, so it will then take over the work itself. He adds: 'Sometimes this involves looking at the mind and the emotions as well.'

Renzo talks of the body fondly, almost like an artist. When speaking of the role of connective tissue, which is where he says my inflammation is lodged, he describes it as a 'passive' tissue changing its shape, like a fishing net. The size of the catch (the strain or injury) it has to hold in its mesh will dictate its shape: either bulging from a heavy load, or close-webbed from a light one. He also describes it as lying in the body in layers, one layer of which has the job of carrying the body's 'memorisation process', the memory of old wounds.

He tells me my own personal fishing net has been stretched way beyond its natural shape for far too long, carrying in its overstrained fibres some big catch from long ago: 'The body is courageous too,' he says. 'It has held you all this time. It has not let you fall.'

I listen to this, for my mind is receptive at last to Renzo's way of describing the body. But trust, that most fragile of nets, still needs more time and repair and I remain quiet, still, about what I've been learning in the armchair.

I've treated my body like the enemy, worked it hard, believed it to be suspect, a possible deceiver rather than a trustworthy and necessary friend.

My body is something which has got me into trouble, even from the age of three or four. It is where God watched me for signs of badness. It is where my pain has occurred. It has been the place of restraint. I have thought of my body and my head, or my mind, as separate, with the mind being the boss, and the body the dumb servant. I've not integrated the two, but my ideas are changing, as are my pains. No work yet, no tennis, but no Big Guns either, no electric shocks, no vice. Many small pains, but otherwise, all is relatively peaceful on the home front.

I'm still cautious, though. Renzo's an osteopath. What I know about myself comes from my work with an analyst. The two are different. Gifted and intuitive though Renzo is, his training, his work, is on the body. My mind is my own business. I continue to ask him about the techniques he is using on me.

On the *physical* front, he says he is carrying on the

work of trying to release tensions and thereby lowering the extent of inflammation. This is what he has been doing all along. He explains again that inflammation *begins* from tension. Small muscles which keep the vertebrae in place become tense through poor use and through too many unbalanced or repetitive movements and the spine gets thrown slightly 'out'.

The reserve troops then muscle in to try and keep the old soldier, the spine, in its proper alignment, and then they get tense from leaning over in the wrong position, and more reserve troops come in and they get tense too, and so it goes on. The connective tissue holding all this lot together gets more and more stretched – and then inflamed.

Renzo also says he is trying to get a better blood supply and more oxygen to my spine and neck, blood and oxygen being vital food supplies for all of the body, especially muscles:

'There, I have written all over your neck,' he says one day in a satisfied voice.

He has, indeed, been pinching and scrunching and kneading my neck to get good blood rushing into it. He now warns me it will be marked in blood-lines for a few hours, but not to worry, they will disappear without trace.

Wryly I suggest it is a liberty, him using my blood supply to write on my body while my own pen lies dormant at home. Connections are forming, though, as treatment continues, links between the armchair video shows and the couch, between the mind and the body. I am ashamed of how I have treated my body – ordering it around with my bossy mind – and I want the damage to stop. Renzo's regard for the body, and the words he uses to describe it, are seeping into me, the image of the nets, especially: strong; trustworthy; ready to catch, hold, keep me together under the skin of myself.

If the tissues which connect my muscles are like fishing nets, I don't want to strain and hurt them any more. Nor do I want to add work to muscles already burdened from trying to bale me out. But deep in these inner seas, old habits still lurk. If you turned a switch and instantly returned me to normal again, I would be back to my bad old body-denying, workaholic ways within weeks.

There is the small altercation over my feet:

'Your feet are not working,' Renzo says to me one warm day. 'They are not doing their job.'

I feel a bit miffed at this. I have nice feet, and tell him so. He laughs.

'Yes, they look very nice,' he agrees, 'but feet are for standing on. Yours,' he adds, 'are like frozen sculptures. They would look good in an exhibition, but on the end of your body . . . ?'

To prove his point, he gently tries to bend my toes, and I wince in pain.

'The pain is from tension,' he tells me.

Is there a single part of my body I can rely on to be free of tension, I wonder? Head, back, arms, fingers, even my feet are tense. How am I to get out of this cage? Where is the freedom I want so much? It seems to be in a different land, a place I cannot reach. I have the will not to hurt myself any more, yet I can't stand properly, let alone see off bad habits snapping, like sharks, at my nets.

'I don't know what to do,' I say to Renzo. 'Every part of my body seems to be tense.'

'No, no,' he corrects me. 'The tension in the upper part of your body is becoming better. Now what you have to do is listen to the other parts. That is all.'
All!

The more I come to like and understand my body, the more like a monster I feel. It has done nothing to deserve what I am doing to it, yet I cannot let go of whatever is keeping me tense still.

It has been fifteen months. I have gone from longing to a place so far beyond it, I can no longer see myself or know the world I have gone to – and still I am awash. Brave muscles and lashings of nets haven't stopped me drifting too deep for safety.

During my years with the *Mail*, in what now seems like a previous lifetime, I had once swum with dolphins. Now I remember a fragment of a dream: a dolphin having difficulty breathing. The animal is alone in a huge ocean trying to swim to shore before it drowns from not being able to take air into its body.
Alone, all at sea, I fear I will not make it to shore.

The day following my visit to Renzo, I'm on the

phone. A friend has rung for a chat, and I am all ears, hanging on her every word. I then become aware of what's happening to my breathing. It's so shallow, it has almost stopped. I seem to be breathing from the neck up, from the chin up even, and am almost holding my breath while I listen, as if it's wrong to breathe while someone else is speaking.

It's how I breathe – or don't breathe – when I work, I realise: bits of air held on to, not released till the next idea, the next sentence, the next bit of light at the end of the tunnel.

The dream fragment of the struggling dolphin comes back to me, as does something else, the childhood instruction: 'Listen to me when I'm talking to you, child. Look at me. Don't fidget.' I remember how I wanted to disappear rather than look in either my father's or Nellie's X-ray eyes. I believe I must have been holding my breath for a long time.

On my next visit to Renzo I ask him to show me some simple breathing exercises:

'I've read about proper breathing,' I say, 'but you're never sure if you've got it quite right.'

Renzo looks puzzled:

'You say you've done yoga all these years? You did not learn breathing?' he asks in a perplexed voice.

I have the decency to look shamefaced. I'd taken up yoga years ago. I now realise I had managed to practise even this most peaceful of exercises like army drill, only more slowly.

'Um, I think we should forget the yoga,' I mumble. 'I think you'll find I was doing it in a tense way.'

He gives me some simple exercises, but also warns me not to overdo them: 'The air will come in and out of your body without you trying too hard,' he says. Then he tells me his centipede story.

One day, a centipede is sitting in the garden minding her own business, having a nice time in the sun, when a worm comes along and starts chatting.

'My, what a wonderful lot of legs you have,' the worm says admiringly. 'Goodness, dozens of them. But tell me something, with all those legs, how do you work out which one to put forward first?'

The centipede is flummoxed. It's a question she doesn't know the answer to and the more she thinks about it, the more she can't find the answer, and the more she can't find the answer, the more she stays stuck, rooted to the spot. The question proves the death of her, for she never walks again.

Shortly after this, I stop keeping the pain notebook. I close it up and shove it in the filing cabinet. Most days I still have small pains in my neck, head, shoulders, arms and hands, but they are not big, incapacitating ones. In any case, there are too many of them to count, probably as many as there are legs on a centipede.

Chapter Twenty-Eight

∽

KEEP NETS (*FOR KEEPING FISH ALIVE*)

Instead of the pain notebook, I begin a new one, a beautiful, leather-bound, soft grey writing book with finely-marked lines. It's as wide as an A4 sheet of paper lying sideways. It's something you would open with ceremony and write in slowly. So, new work begins. The book's feel, shape, its soft colour and smooth pages satisfy me enough that a few sentences at a time will do, as they have to. I had not imagined anything less than a thousand words a day could be called work. Now, it's clear I can't hurry the words.

To make sure I don't spend too long with a pen in my hand, I set aside time slots: two ten-minute ones in the morning and two in the afternoon. When there are no repercussions, I increase them to six a day – a whole hour. There I stop. Better to inch forward slowly than be flung all the way back to the start. At the first sign of a small ache, I learn to put down the pen and imagine I have other important things to see to.

As this is happening, connections which have been waiting to be noticed are seen at last. The Big Guns are in my mind: my father and his God one steel-eyed threat; Nellie the other. A long time ago their purpose was to make me who they wanted me to be, their version of a child instead of my own. Years later, their regime in my body has almost destroyed me, but not quite.

'Are you still travelling all the way to Maidstone?' some people ask me.

'Yes,' I reply. 'The treatment is working.'

'But surely there are good osteopaths in London? Why go all that way?'

I can't begin to explain.

The conversations with Renzo continue around the body. We have touched on my frozen feet; my head, which houses my too-fierce mind; my neck, which he has written on, as I had done first. I had put it on the line – for work and to defend myself. Day after day I had stuck my neck out far beyond safety to fight giants, produce books and stare at computer screens.

Then there are the shoulders, the baggage carriers which have shouldered so much for so long – fear, worry, a lifetime of carrying round precious cargo from when I was too young – the weight of memory. Slabs of Africa, coffin nightmares, Egyptian fans, I thought I would lose them if I put them down and they would disappear, taking me with them. The person who would help me unpack the events of my life as I moved from one place to another was missing. No one kept my past for me, so my child's work was to hold onto it.

If you trace the history of a life through muscles, there are too many goliaths in my story, too many wars, too much weight of responsibility on my shoulders. With all the changes of school, language wasn't easy for me either and I hoarded it clumsily: jagged thoughts; rocks; boulders; slingfuls of words.

'The story of your life, your history, is written in your body,' Renzo says one day.
So he knows.

He says that although it is difficult to give a strict geography of emotions in the body, he nevertheless associates a bad problem in the cervical spine, the neck region, with fear and anger. He says:

'The body's way of reacting to a strong emotion is linked with the shoulders. When you have a deep fear, you bring your shoulders and arms up to protect your head. If there are strong emotions, you bring certain contractions in the muscles. It can be active, like wanting to punch someone with anger, and it can also be in the connective tissue. In the layers of connective tissues in the body, one layer has a function of memorisation of traumas. I do not mean only physical traumas. As I understand the body, the connective tissue has an important part to play in memorising what happened to us during all of our life.'
So the nets were keeping the narrative all along.

Renzo talks about the 'fear' which he says my body has so eloquently told him of. He reminds me he had asked for a chest X-ray after first seeing me because he thought there was something wrong with my lungs (which there was not).

'It was so obvious you were protecting your chest in a very, very strong way as if you had been afraid for a long time. Your shoulders were anterior [leaning forwards]. There was so much muscle tension there, it was preventing the bone from settling back. All of this was so, so strong, as if you were protecting something very personal around your heart.' He adds:

'Then you ask me about breathing, and I am amazed. I see you have not let air freely in and out of your lungs, perhaps for most of your life. That is why I thought there was something wrong with them. You did it through fear, and through trying to protect where the hurt was.'

End of lesson.

If the stories of our lives are told in our bodies, my struggle with the towering giants of my childhood – and with my mother's love being rationed through her illness – has been recorded. Too painful to bear consciously, it was stored in my 'trunk'.

The 'forgotten' muscles which my mind had refused to remember were, indeed, the ones around my beleaguered and frightened heart. My refusal and neglect of the tension in this region was my wish for the pain in my heart not to be felt. I ignored this part of me for fear the truth would stop my heartbeat, take my breath away.

But the body *is* courageous, and had soldiered on. While, as an adult, I turned my back and refused to remember what my childhood self had kept safely stored for me, it had dutifully carried on recording the events of my life. But the strain was great, and its memory nets had stretched over the years under the weight of what my mind could not or would not carry. The strain had eventually '*told*' on them, and they had begun to fray. They had then spoken to me directly, contacted the boss. They were angry and inflamed with the injustice of what they had had to bear while I carried on my life regardless.

There had been grief before, so I thought, but it's a monsoon now. Hours of rain, days, weeks of it, thick curtains of tears dampening pages, splashing my lap.

In my body, the place where I am hurting, the flood brings ease. The keep nets which have held the terror and rage, which have stretched and strained, are floating again, drifting easily, 'affected', now that I am, in a different way. I recall the dream, in Sharjah, of objects from the dolls' house floating on a calm sea. The picture, now, in the armchair, is of a child again, a four-year-old girl bending forwards to write something – a person full of pencils.

As a growing child, keeping pencils wherever I could, I hid them even at night. I slept with a pencil and bit of paper under my pillow rather than leaving them by the side of the bed where they might be stolen. The person who might have done this was my father. He'd taken them from me when he locked me up as a small child and, as I grew to seven or eight years old, he would mockingly snatch them out of my hand. Yet, stubbornly, tenaciously, I kept them with me.

There was a pencil and paper in my dressing-gown pocket on my bed-time walks between Number 77 and 85 in Wales. Wherever my pencil and paper were, there was I.

I must have felt the need to bear witness, for my identity depended on it. If my story was being written down, then the details of it had not buried me, nor left me mute and invisible. While I could write I could be heard behind the bars of my cage or the lid of my coffin.

I have often thought of Renzo as a human stethoscope. He seems to be able to 'hear' things with his hands, and also, sometimes, with his ear when he leans his head close to my body. When he works in this way with his ear near my back, chest or shoulder, I find it reassuring, a signal, perhaps, of how closely he is paying attention. When, once, I ask why he is doing this, he says he is listening.

I know now what he means, for my body has been telling him something. It had something important to say, and somebody had to listen after all these years. If, however, he had said he was reading I might have seen the last bit of the picture earlier. For if the stories of our lives are written or told in our bodies, I need not have worried for dear life about my pencil and paper being taken. For the details had been stored, my body the paper – the book – the words were written on.

They were there, in blood-lines, in skin maps, in feet sculptures, in arcing muscles and in the memory webs of stretched nets. They were stored there waiting for the woman who lived among them to be ready to read what was so close to her that she couldn't see. When it looked as if she would never attend, that she would live a life blind to herself, the alarm was raised.

By the time Renzo and I finally finish working together, two years have passed since the Big Guns first let me know there was a war on. Two years after the first hostilities were declared, my muscles have at last released their grip on my shoulder bones, air is coming more freely in and out of my chest, and I have begun to walk distances, cook for people and return to life again. More than anything else, I am able to begin sustained and serious work.

I take it slowly though. When he'd told me I would need patience, I had not thought, in my wildest imagination, I would be able to find as much as I have. I would have said it was impossible for someone as impatient as me to lie down four times in the course of a morning's work to help ease my shoulders and spine and, more important than the lying-down itself, to learn not to resent it.

But perhaps essential lessons have at last been

'heard' from that central intelligence source, my own body. Catching on to its messages of distress has taken a long time, and has changed the set of my mind as well as the shape of my bones. Now, when I want to push myself again, to do too much, I keep on thinking, deeply, of the patience of those nets, and how, despite everything, all the abuse, they have held.

I am getting well again and the knowledge slowly creeps up on me as I begin to trust. The first outward sign of this is my willingness to believe I can physically leave the house I have lived in for more than a decade and move somewhere else. It still takes other people to tell me progress is being made, that a year previously I couldn't easily lift a knife or fork, let alone have the stamina to move house.

Installed in a new home, I am recovered enough to be leaning on words again in my mind, although not with my body. For I sit upright in the study this time, head erect, shoulders relaxed, feet flat on the floor.

I stay calm, grounded, as, page by page, this, the new book, begins. When it pulls me forward towards the screen I slowly lean back again. My mind can go on, but my body must stay back. This mustn't run away with me.

'Patience' has been the password, and I have sat still for enough time now to see why: impatience from a long way back has been one of the root causes of my affliction. Not just ordinary impatience, but the extra- ordinary will of a child on a bedroom shelf trying to punch a hole in Time and propel herself into the future.

When 'tomorrow' arrived, she did the same thing over again. I don't blame her for it. She had a long way to travel to be grown enough to wrestle her life back from those who tried to steal it from her.

As our parting draws near I at last tell Renzo a little about what I am writing – a personal account of the history of an incapacity, the long journey back to the source of a crime, a kind of physiological whodunnit. At our final meeting I give him a copy of my last book, the one on grief, and ask him something:

'Has anyone else ever tested your patience as much as I have?'

'No,' he says with a warm smile. Then, with a flourish, he adds in his usual French English: 'You are – how do you say? – the first.'

Chapter Twenty-Nine

෨ᵹ

MY GRANDMOTHER'S SHOES

When I was nine, an uncle helped me make a puppet. We wanted to make the spine out of cotton reels but, searching through my aunt's sewing box, there weren't enough empty ones for the job. A few were heading that way with only a small amount of thread, and my uncle decided to hijack them. It's my earliest remembered experience of an adult breaking household laws. I was staying on my own for a while with this aunt and uncle outside Bulawayo, and most concerned not to offend them. I was therefore amazed, alarmed and delighted at my uncle's domestic misrule.

'Sit where you are,' he told me. Tiptoeing off, his shoulders shaking as he chuckled with the mischief of it all, he returned a few minutes later with some stiff cardboard. He cut a few notches in it, and we wound the thread from the almost-empty cotton reels into those.

When my aunt caught us at it, I was further astonished and delighted when my ally and hero won the battle on our behalf:

'Oh don't be silly,' he told my chiding aunt. 'It's only a bit of cotton, and it's all back there, tidy. Look, we haven't messed up your sewing box. Now, where were we?'

We tried threading first wire, then, eventually, thick elastic through the reels in order to keep them in place on top of each other, but at the right, flexible tension. They needed to bend and bounce for the puppet to dance. It danced and rolled around the stage that night at the concert my girl cousin and I held for the grown-ups, and my uncle clapped the loudest.

I had once thought my body was un-remembering. Not so. The return of my cotton-reel spine with its cheerful flexibility is like a homecoming. A combination of Renzo's ministrations, Alexander Technique lessons and patience has prevailed.

There are changes too. The months of enforced stillness have produced a slight 'formality'. Physically, my body's straighter, my shoulders have dropped, settling back to a more comfortable position and, although there's no weight gained, I've expanded. I'm a centimetre taller, slightly broader, 'sculptured' feet half a size bigger. No longer trapped by bars, I inhabit all the space inside me, breathing in and out to the limits of my skin.

Being calmer, it's easier to see what's happening around me now, to wait for things, watch and listen. I used to be a woman with too much of the future in me to wait for anything. Sometimes I feel like someone in charge of a body again and not an integrated whole. But it's not one-way traffic. If my head decides my body needs a break from typing, it's because it's listening, not playing boss.

It's a kinder authority and my slow return to tennis is reward for the hundreds of days of exercise to keep muscles and limbs mobile. Spontaneity: what I most enjoy. No time to worry who's in charge on a tennis court, only watch the ball and hit it.

At business meetings it's different. I've forgotten something. I can't speak the way I used to and struggle to be heard. Other people's strong, capable voices overwhelm me and I almost stammer in attempts to speak up. But I must surface from the steep dive into myself, find my voice again from where it has been soundless under the sea.

From this deep place I remember the armchair picture of the girl with the bird beating its wings in her chest while she tries to hold on to words which are flying away. I take on chairing a committee, nervous of what once I did with ease. There's a long way to swim up.

So that's it, then? The story finished?

Not quite.

Someone had to grieve in our family. My parents

wouldn't, couldn't, do it. Passed on, unwrapped, it's been with me from the beginning, like the rage and anger woven in with my past: 'Why haven't you grieved for your childhood?' a friend once asked.

Answer: Because I couldn't feel it. My childhood seemed like a story which might have happened to somebody else. As my parents had done, I felt nothing to cry for. It wasn't until I dived under the wreckage from the armchair and found so much kept, the vast world of a buried childhood, not gone, nor lost, but here, that grief could begin – through pictures as well as words.

Children are baggage carriers for the dreams and nightmares of the people they grow up among and my father's biggest nightmare was Dresden. In the small hours of Valentine's Day 1945, he took part in a raid of first British and then Allied forces, who flattened the city in wave after wave of bombs.

To pulverise a civilian population was a controversial decision. As a way of building Anglo-German relationships after the War, the British Government engaged in a contorted act of diplomacy and contrition. They flew some of the Lancaster crews over to Dresden, so the men could be seen to witness at first hand what they'd done. My father was one of these people, and he was faced with a dilemma he couldn't cope with. It wasn't in his moral repertoire to have done this. Religion was in his life since childhood, a punitive old-Testament religion, an eye for an eye – but not this.

I believe the precious thing I broke in childhood was the Dresden Doll my father brought back at the end of the War, not in his arms for, like the blue lamp, no such object existed, but in his mind.

If I would be a perfect child, if he could make me into that, with God's help, then the world would be whole again, his part in Dresden redeemed.

I wasn't. The world remained broken.

The grief running through my father's life was depression: his mother's; his father's; and, eventually, as a child of depression, his own. For a long time it was my grief too, stealing my vitality, 'robbing me blind' as I searched in the dark along motorways, scanning people's windows for what I couldn't have – a clear view from the inside, ordinary ease. There are days when I'm locked in like this still, when I don't have the power to break the glass: a lack of affection.

Other days, like a light switched on, there's plenty of clear space in my mind, a large circular hallway where depression is held back. I have a sense of what's been built over the years – a vantage point – somewhere to see and save a life.

The vanishings and losses I remember now are not from childhood. They're from later. They come from my adult travelling, taking the form of not being able to hold on to my days, the good ones that is. At the end of a trip away, I feel the place I visited has died.

On good days, I can still travel and hold on to things: visualise Africa; know the scent of it weeks later. On bad ones I can no more imagine Newcastle or Scotland, let alone a Saharan desert or Tanzanian plain.

I lose places. They go dark on me or, as I've come to realise, I go dark on them, like a light going out. Then I remember Egypt and putting my Welsh grandparents out of my mind because I didn't know whether or not they were real. Standing under the fan, clinging on to my mother's legs, I 'killed' them because I didn't know if I'd imagined them or not.

My father is churchless by now. I do not know why, but we have begun to talk. Calmer, the thunderous moods of his depressions are less prolonged, but he's lost. He's rung to say he still can't read. Or at least he can, but he doesn't know which books. He's tried opening ones I suggested, but they don't make sense. They're strangers to him, and he's afraid to go to the library because he doesn't know where to look or what to ask for.

Which is why we're here, in the library, taking down books. He's shrunk over the years, from six foot, perhaps an inch or two gone, and I've grown through my spine straightening out of its terror. So we're level among the shelves, standing with books in our hands, me showing him how the system works, where to go for help, taking him to sections where he might find what he's looking for. I don't think it will work. After a lifetime of turning his back on words, they're unlikely to speak to him now.

But I'm pleased to try.

I haven't looked my father in the eye for as long as I can remember. Now we stand, face to face, and perhaps he can see me at last, for he asks what I do with my life, says he's interested and wants to know.

The first wounding was in my eye, in my place of knowing what was real or not, in my view of myself and my ability to form good judgement. I was told I was a bad, wrong child. Fighting for the light, I tried to find a different perspective.

The second wound was in my heart. From a young age, I grieved for my parents' unhappiness and the badness in our family. As I grew older, I built a breast-plate of muscles to try and hide my hurt, to defend myself.

The third wound was in my spine, like Nellie's, bent inside me – a physical curve smaller than her deformity, but there to stop me growing straight. More crippling than this, mistrust of my backbone and resolve – a lack of nerve and belief.

Children whose stories are listened to thrive. You can see it happening to them as they grow by the word. A problem with stories and words runs in our family. I learn the extent of it after reclaiming my mother. Speaking Welsh to her for the first time on the phone, she's different: stronger, more thoughtful and attentive.

She tells me Welsh was the language she thought and dreamed in most of her young married life. It was the language she called out in, startling the staff of an East African hospital when my brother was born. Yet her mother-in-law – and my father too – overpowered her in English, a language she couldn't defend herself in.

Her cards begin to arrive soon after this.

The first one shows a Pembroke coastal scene. Inside, my mother writes in the language of her childhood, and tells me things about her past, about being kept away from school to bring up her younger brothers and sisters while my grandmother played the piano. She was made to cook Sunday dinners, to shop, clean and put the other children to bed while Bessie lived for her music. 'I was a most unloved girl,' she writes in Welsh.

As if to make up for those empty airmails from Africa, my mother sends postcards from Wales every week or so, carefully chosen, and when there's a gap, she'll ring to say she's on the lookout for a nice one.

One weekend, I treat her and my aunt and uncle, who have given me hearth space, to a night out in London. We go to an opera at Covent Garden and, for the fun of it, dress up. It's warm, and we stroll around. My mother is wearing green again, a green blouse, with a floor-length skirt.

As we come into the open area where the buskers play, it's almost empty, a clear space in inner London under a blue evening sky. A lone Irish fiddler starts up with a jig, and before I know what has happened, my mother has me by the waist, and is swirling me round the piazza. Round and round we dance, taking up the square as we gather pace, flying along with the music. When it stops, there's loud clapping and, looking round, breathless, there are hundreds of people gathered, all enjoying the dance.

With Chris, my brother, I've always been close. While he's lost much of his young childhood to memory losses and family blanks, I've kept some of the stories for him: the elephant in the garden; the way we closed ranks and ganged up on our parents over creatures in the house, over bedtimes and over scoldings and rows. We took each other's part.

There was better fortune for him with schooling. He stayed in Cardiff from an eight-year-old onwards and had ten continuous years of education and the chance to settle, form relationships and keep the thread of memory safe. Firm friendships were made, and this part of his history is safe.

I have four favourite pictures from the family album. The first belongs to my inner camera: a small girl sits on a kitchen table. Finger and thumb in the air, she's measuring the size of naughtiness that might be allowed in her over-watched days if God and her father would only be reasonable. Negotiating for all she is worth, she's exercising a child's prerogative to try, no matter what the size, shape or strength of the opposition.

The second picture is the snapshot of my mother shielding her eyes against a hot desert sun and looking calm and unassailable in the light and space around her.

The third is Chris as a three-year-old in Tanzania. He's playing, and holds a rock which he's about to throw – but he's already on to the next thing, as if the rock's gone from his hand. You can see it behind his eyes. 'What's after this? How much playing, throwing, running, pushing, swimming, kicking, jumping up and down can I do?'

The fourth picture is of my mother and father in evening dress on board the *Pretoria Castle* in 1959. It's before the dance, and they both seem out of their depth and nervous, he no less than she. The picture says he would run if he could.

It's three years since the Big Guns began their salvos in me and my body has survived against my fear it wouldn't take the strain of resuming work. A small pain in the early days had me hurrying to rest in case it was the first warning of being sent back for a prolonged spell in the armchair. Would the disabling vice return to stop this? Would the story be stolen again when I'd got this far? It's not until now, when I know the book is safe, almost done, that there's the dream:

Friends are gathered round in a big house, people from Africa, smiling faces, activity. But I have to hide something in a small bit of paper, like a chewing-gum wrapper: white powder – an illicit drug?

Then, policemen are coming on a routine search and I wrap the chewing-gum packet in masses of silver paper, but it's too bulky, so I unwrap it again, and leave it as it is. The two policemen are young, friendly, in plain clothes. They easily find the white powder and aren't concerned. It's normal, they say, for people to break the law a little.

So this book is allowed.

Its story is one of a girl being trapped – in a trunk and by too many pairs of critical eyes – who grows into a woman on the run. But with claustrophobia on the inside, she lives in a box wherever she goes. Therapy slows her down, opens her up a little, makes her think, but it takes being incapacitated to stop her flight from the past. Friends have warned her:

'You drive yourself too hard. What are you running from? *Who* are you running from?'

They get nowhere. She's hell bent.

The story told in my body is that of a child, as children do, trying to hold on to what is hers while people try and take it from her. What she wants to hold on to is her version of the truth – herself. This is what she has, the sum of it, and is what she can hope to know. In the tug-o-war between my two fathers and myself I was a child who wouldn't let go of my end of the rope. I would have my own words. I would not have theirs.

In any difficult family, someone has to carry the burden, pick up the tab, and that's what I did. But a child who doesn't wish to become mad, who wants to have her life and to describe it the way she chooses, may use the body to house her story. She will do this, I think, in pictures as well as words.

Hell doesn't live in my body any more. Fear and occasional panic still do and it's work — and work again — to contain them. I spend a long time talking to my terror, in a train of all places, on an eight-hour journey back from Aberdeen. Usually uncontentious ground for me, trains, but this is new rolling stock: super-sealed; air conditioned; electronically operated doors, no opening windows, not a handle in sight. You take the space and air they give you and I don't like it.

While we're moving I'm all right. It's when the train stops between stations and the air conditioning fails on a warm summer's day that the panic starts. I try to be calm, tell myself I've been here before. Stay still. Hold on till it passes. But a panic attack is like a house caving in and it's on you, over you, before you see it happening — a collapse of perspective.

The world tilts away again, growing out of size, and I'm in thrall to a four-year-old with the lid of the trunk coming down on her head, words flying out of her, terrified she'll be all gone and there'll be no girl left. Physically she grips me: palpitations; a big bird's fluttering heartbeat takes over mine; tension in my stomach; bars across my chest; moist palms; a dry throat and the urge to run out of my skin from fear. Panic ascending, the world around me pales as my eyes 'white out' colour in the fields and sky outside. I blink carefully, for it seems I might go blind with the effort of holding onto myself.

With the train moving again, slowly I walk a little. It would soothe me to put my head outside an open window and meet a cool breeze. But the panic has happened because the window isn't there – at least not to be opened. Another trap from childhood: being shut behind glass, away from life, unable to break out.

The train speeding up, reason tells me I will not spend the rest of my days sealed in like this. Speaking to myself in my mind, using words, saying them slowly, I breathe the walls of my adult life out again, push them back up. The beating and fluttering in my chest subside: 'It's only glass,' I say, 'and it won't be there much longer.'

You're supposed not to write stories like this one. To protect the old guard, the status quo, you're meant to keep the lid on the trunk, the bung in the glass bottle, the door to what goes on in families closed. But if you do, the past will tower over and bury the future for ever.

Nellie returns at this point in the story. With only a page or so to go, the presence of my English grand-mother in my days and nights is overwhelming. She's young, around twenty, and trying urgently to tell me something, but she has no voice.

In a dream I'm in the nineteenth century, looking for a path through some woods and in danger of losing my way. Nellie is ahead of me and shows me where to go – along a track where brightly coloured guinea fowl with golden neck feathers roam freely. The path leads to a large comfortable house where dinner will be served at eight. Looking down at my feet, I find I'm wearing Nellie's heavy lace-up shoes.

Waking, I sense I've lived with a crooked grand-mother inside me for years. While her shoes remind me of this, they also speak of sturdiness, and I believe the dream tells me my feelings about the people who've formed my life have changed. No longer the Big Guns of my childhood, my father and Nellie have human proportions by this time. I've found a different way.

For the first time in a decade, I travel in a tube, just one stop from Highbury and Islington to King's Cross – with a friend. Then I do it again on my own. I've been in a lift seven or eight times, first of all with someone, then solo.

So who – what – is the life-saver in the end: the body; the mind; the child; the therapist; the friend who makes me dive deeper for the words on this page; the osteopath with his intuition and respect; or the woman who refuses to give in?

It's a place, I believe, for all of these. At the bottom of any story, there's a place of memory and resistance: a night-time seabed; an underground cathedral; a factory full of children; a circular hallway; a come-to-life photograph; a child's den.

At the bottom of every life there's a story.

I was bound to be seized, it seems to me, and made to sit still, for my body had worked hard for decades to keep a history safe. The original wound was in the mind and the body paid the penalty for what the mind couldn't face. It then itself suffered the breakdown the mind could not afford to have: grief and affection were a long time coming.

When the mind was ready, at last, to shoulder its share of the burden of knowledge of a life, memory was intact and a child's buried words were given their chance to speak. They had been stored in muscles, written in blood-lines: a history kept in a cinema show of pictures, images and dreams. Having held on to it for so long, the body was inflamed and angry.

Through Big Guns, Iron Fingers, manacles and vices, it captured a woman, sat her down in a chair and said: 'Look. Listen. I have something to say.'